NAVIGATING

HERNIA

A Comprehensive Guide to Prevention, Treatment, and Recovery

BY

MARIA JOSEPHINE

TABLE OF CONTENT

INTRODUCTION

When I first encountered the word "hernia," it sounded like a mysterious and somewhat intimidating medical term. Like many of you, I had questions swirling in my mind. What exactly is a hernia? Is it something I should be worried about? How does it affect the body, and what can be done about it? Through my journey of learning and understanding hernias, I realized that this is a topic shrouded in myths and misconceptions, often leaving people either overly anxious or too dismissive of its seriousness.

So, what exactly is a hernia? Simply put, a hernia occurs when an organ or tissue pushes through a weak spot in the surrounding muscle or connective tissue. Imagine a balloon squeezing through a small tear in a tire. It's not always painful, and sometimes you might not even notice it at first, but as it progresses, it can become a significant health issue. Hernias are more common than you might think, and they can happen to anyone, regardless of age or gender.

Why is understanding hernias crucial for overall health? Because knowledge is power. When we understand what a hernia is, what causes it, and how it can affect our body, we are better equipped to prevent it, recognize the signs early, and seek appropriate treatment. Ignoring a hernia can lead to complications that could have been easily avoided with timely intervention. On the flip side, overreacting without proper knowledge can lead to unnecessary stress and anxiety.

This book is about empowerment. I want to provide you with the information you need to take control of your health when it comes to hernias. Whether you're someone who's trying to prevent a hernia, living with one, or recovering from treatment, my goal is to offer practical advice grounded in both medical expertise and real-life experiences.

We'll explore the anatomy of hernias, the causes, and risk factors, and how to spot the early warning signs. I'll guide you through the various treatment options available and what to expect during recovery. But more than that, I want to share strategies for prevention, because prevention is always better than cure. Through personal stories, case studies, and the latest research, we'll demystify hernias together.

So, let's dive in and equip ourselves with the knowledge needed to tackle hernias head-on, ensuring a healthier, more informed life. Welcome to your comprehensive guide to understanding, managing, and overcoming hernias.

Chapter 1: Demystifying Hernias

What is a Hernia?

At its core, a hernia is a medical condition that occurs when an organ or tissue pushes through a weak spot or tear in the muscle or connective tissue that normally holds it in place. This protrusion can happen in various parts of the body, and while some hernias are relatively harmless and painless, others can lead to significant discomfort and serious health complications if not properly managed.

To fully understand hernias, it's important to explore the different types that exist. Each type of hernia is classified based on its location and the underlying causes that lead to its formation. Let's delve into the most common types:

Inguinal Hernia

An inguinal hernia is the most common type, accounting for approximately 75% of all hernia cases. It occurs when a portion of the intestine or fatty tissue pushes through the inguinal canal, which is located in the groin area. This type predominantly affects men due to the natural weakness in the abdominal wall where the spermatic cord passes through. Women can also experience inguinal hernias, though it is less common.

Symptoms may include a visible bulge in the groin, discomfort or pain, especially when bending over, lifting, or coughing. In severe cases, it can lead to strangulation, where the blood supply to the herniated tissue is cut off, requiring immediate surgical intervention.

Femoral Hernia

Femoral hernias are similar to inguinal hernias but occur lower in the groin, just below the inguinal ligament. They are more common in women, particularly those who are pregnant or obese. This type of hernia can be hard to detect initially, as the bulge may not be immediately noticeable.

Like inguinal hernias, femoral hernias can lead to complications if left untreated, including obstruction or strangulation of the intestines. Prompt diagnosis and treatment are crucial.

Umbilical Hernia

An umbilical hernia happens when part of the intestine or other tissues protrude through the abdominal wall near the navel (umbilicus). This type of hernia is common in infants, especially those born prematurely, as the abdominal wall muscles haven't fully developed. However, adults, particularly those who are overweight or have undergone multiple pregnancies, can also develop umbilical hernias.

In infants, umbilical hernias often close on their own within the first few years of life. In adults, surgical repair may be necessary, especially if the hernia becomes painful or enlarges.

Hiatal Hernia

A hiatal hernia is somewhat different from the other types because it involves the stomach pushing up through the diaphragm into the chest cavity. This type is further classified into sliding and paraesophageal hernias. Sliding hiatal hernias are the most common and typically do not cause significant issues. However, paraesophageal hernias, where a part of the stomach pushes beside the esophagus, can lead to more severe problems like strangulation.

Hiatal hernias are often associated with gastroesophageal reflux disease (GERD), causing symptoms such as heartburn, chest pain, and difficulty swallowing. Lifestyle changes, medications, and sometimes surgery are used to manage this type of hernia.

Incisional Hernia

An incisional hernia can develop at the site of a previous surgical incision in the abdominal wall. After surgery, the area around the incision may remain weak, creating a potential point for herniation, especially if the wound doesn't heal properly or if there is excessive strain on the area.

These hernias are more likely to occur in people who are obese, those who have undergone multiple abdominal surgeries, or individuals who engage in strenuous physical activity soon after surgery. Repair usually involves surgical intervention to strengthen the weakened area.

Understanding the different types of hernias is crucial because each type has unique characteristics, risk factors, and treatment approaches. As we move forward in this guide, we'll explore these aspects in more detail, helping you identify symptoms early and seek the appropriate care to prevent complications. Whether you're dealing with a hernia personally or supporting someone who is, having this foundational knowledge is the first step in demystifying this common health condition.

Anatomy of a Hernia

To truly understand hernias, it's essential to delve into the anatomy of the human body and identify the regions most susceptible to this condition. Hernias occur when there is a weakness or defect in the muscular or fascial layer that usually keeps organs and tissues in place. Let's explore the anatomical regions prone to hernias and understand how hernias develop in these areas.

The Anatomical Regions Prone to Hernias

1. **Inguinal Region (Groin Area)**
The inguinal region is the most common site for hernias, particularly for inguinal hernias. The inguinal canal, through which structures such as the spermatic cord in men and the round ligament in women pass, is a naturally weak area in the lower abdominal wall. Over time, or due to strain, this area can weaken further, leading to hernia formation.

2. **Femoral Canal**
Located just below the inguinal ligament, the femoral canal is another weak spot, especially in women. This canal allows the femoral artery, vein, and nerve to pass through, but it can also become a point of herniation, leading to femoral hernias.

3. Umbilical Region

The umbilical area is a potential weak spot because it was once the site of the umbilical cord attachment during fetal development. In infants, the abdominal muscles surrounding the umbilicus may not fully close after birth, leading to umbilical hernias. In adults, factors like obesity, multiple pregnancies, and abdominal strain can lead to the development of umbilical hernias.

4. Hiatal Region (Diaphragm)

The diaphragm has an opening, the esophageal hiatus, through which the esophagus passes. Weakness in this area can lead to hiatal hernias, where part of the stomach pushes up into the chest cavity. This is a unique hernia type because it involves the diaphragm, which separates the thoracic and abdominal cavities.

5. Incisional Sites

Any previous surgical site on the abdominal wall can be prone to incisional hernias. After surgery, the healing process might leave the area weaker than the rest of the abdominal wall, making it vulnerable to herniation, especially under increased pressure.

How Hernias Develop

Hernias develop when there is an increase in intra-abdominal pressure combined with a weakness in the abdominal wall or fascia. This pressure can force part of an organ or tissue to push through the weak spot, forming a hernia. Here's how this process typically unfolds:

1. Weakness in the Abdominal Wall

- **Congenital Weakness:** Some individuals are born with weak areas in their abdominal wall, making them more susceptible to hernias. For example, the inguinal canal is a naturally weak point, especially in men.

• **Acquired Weakness:** Over time, factors such as aging, injury, or previous surgery can weaken the muscles and connective tissue, creating potential sites for hernias.

2. **Increased Intra-Abdominal Pressure**

• **Physical Strain:** Activities like heavy lifting, straining during bowel movements, or persistent coughing can increase abdominal pressure.

• **Obesity and Pregnancy:** These conditions can also elevate intra-abdominal pressure over time, contributing to hernia development.

• **Chronic Conditions:** Diseases that cause chronic coughing, sneezing, or difficulty urinating can also contribute to the formation of hernias.

3. **Protrusion of Tissues**
When the pressure within the abdomen exceeds the strength of the weakened area, tissues such as the intestines, fatty tissue, or even parts of the stomach can push through, forming a visible bulge or causing discomfort.

4. **Progression**
Initially, the herniated tissue may retract when lying down or with gentle manipulation. However, over time, the opening can enlarge, making the hernia more noticeable and potentially leading to complications like incarceration or strangulation.

Understanding the anatomy and mechanics behind hernia formation helps in both preventing and managing this condition. Recognizing the regions most prone to hernias and the factors that increase intra-abdominal pressure can empower individuals to take proactive measures, such as strengthening core muscles and avoiding unnecessary strain, which we will explore further in later chapters.

Chapter 2: Causes and Risk Factors

Genetic and Lifestyle Factors

Hernias can result from a complex interplay between genetic predisposition and lifestyle choices. Understanding these factors can help identify who might be at greater risk and offer insights into preventive strategies. Let's examine the role of genetics and how lifestyle choices contribute to hernia development.

The Role of Genetics

Some people are born with a higher susceptibility to hernias due to inherited traits or congenital weaknesses in the body's structural integrity. Here's how genetics come into play:

1. **Congenital Weaknesses**

   • **Inguinal Hernias in Infants:** Some infants are born with a condition where the inguinal canal does not close properly, leading to a congenital inguinal hernia. This condition is more common in premature babies, as their bodies haven't fully developed by birth.

   • **Connective Tissue Disorders:** Genetic conditions such as Ehlers-Danlos syndrome or Marfan syndrome can weaken connective tissues, making individuals more prone to hernias.

14

2. **Familial History**

• **Inherited Predisposition:** If hernias are common in your family, you may inherit a predisposition to developing them. This could be due to a shared genetic tendency for weaker abdominal walls or connective tissues.

Understanding these genetic factors highlights the importance of early monitoring and intervention in individuals with a family history of hernias or connective tissue disorders.

How Lifestyle Choices Contribute to Hernia Development

Lifestyle choices significantly influence the likelihood of developing a hernia. Certain behaviors and conditions can increase intra-abdominal pressure or weaken the abdominal wall, contributing to hernia formation. Let's explore the key lifestyle factors:

1. **Physical Strain**

• **Heavy Lifting:** Regularly lifting heavy objects without proper technique can place excessive pressure on the abdominal wall, leading to hernias, especially in the inguinal or incisional regions.

• **Straining During Bowel Movements or Urination:** Chronic constipation or conditions like an enlarged prostate can cause individuals to strain, increasing the risk of hernias over time.

2. **Obesity**

• Excess body weight increases the strain on the abdominal muscles, making them more prone to developing weak spots where hernias can form. This is particularly relevant for umbilical and incisional hernias.

3. Smoking

• Smoking affects tissue strength and impairs healing, weakening the abdominal wall. Chronic coughing associated with smoking also increases abdominal pressure, raising the risk of hernias, especially hiatal hernias.

4. Poor Nutrition

• A diet lacking in essential nutrients, such as proteins and vitamins, can impair tissue repair and overall muscle health, weakening the body's ability to withstand intra-abdominal pressure.

5. Sedentary Lifestyle

• Lack of regular exercise can lead to weakened core muscles, reducing the support they provide to the abdominal wall and increasing the likelihood of hernia development.

6. Pregnancy

• The increased pressure on the abdominal wall during pregnancy can lead to hernias, especially in women who have multiple pregnancies or are carrying multiples (twins, triplets, etc.).

7. Chronic Diseases

• Conditions such as chronic cough (from asthma or COPD), or diseases that cause recurrent vomiting or sneezing, can contribute to the increased pressure in the abdominal cavity, facilitating hernia formation.

Balancing Genetic and Lifestyle Factors

While you can't change your genetic makeup, you can modify lifestyle choices to mitigate the risk of hernia development. By adopting healthier habits, such as maintaining a healthy weight, practicing proper lifting techniques, quitting smoking, and strengthening the core muscles, you can significantly reduce the likelihood of developing a hernia, even if you have a genetic predisposition.

In the next section, we'll explore additional risk factors, including occupational hazards and medical conditions, further expanding on the complex causes of hernias.

Occupational Hazards

Certain jobs and activities can significantly increase the risk of developing hernias due to the physical demands they place on the body. Occupations that involve heavy lifting, repetitive strain, or prolonged periods of standing can put excessive pressure on the abdominal wall and increase intra-abdominal pressure, creating opportunities for hernias to develop. Let's take a closer look at the types of jobs and activities that pose higher risks.

Jobs That Increase Hernia Risk

1. **Manual Laborers**

   • **Construction Workers:** This job often involves lifting heavy materials, operating machinery, and repetitive bending or squatting, which can strain the abdominal muscles.

- **Warehouse Workers:** Tasks such as loading and unloading goods require constant heavy lifting, which increases the risk of hernias, particularly inguinal and incisional types.

2. **Healthcare Workers**

- **Nurses and Caregivers:** Frequently lifting or repositioning patients, especially in long-term care settings, puts healthcare workers at risk of developing hernias.

- **Surgeons and Dental Professionals:** Although not typically associated with heavy lifting, these professionals often stand for long hours, which can increase abdominal pressure and the likelihood of hernia development over time.

3. **Agricultural Workers**

- **Farmers and Landscapers:** Handling heavy equipment, lifting feed or fertilizer bags, and repetitive movements such as bending to plant or harvest crops contribute to hernia risk.

4. **Athletes and Physical Trainers**

- **Weightlifters and Bodybuilders:** The constant heavy lifting, particularly when not done with proper form, can strain the abdominal wall.

- **Professional Athletes:** Sports that involve sudden twists, heavy impacts, or intense abdominal pressure (e.g., football, wrestling) can lead to hernias, especially in the groin area (sports hernias).

5. **Public Safety Workers**

- **Police Officers and Firefighters:** In addition to the physical demands of their jobs, carrying heavy gear and equipment can increase abdominal pressure and the risk of hernias.

• **Military Personnel:** The combination of carrying heavy packs, engaging in strenuous physical activity, and enduring prolonged standing or running can lead to hernias.

Activities That Increase Hernia Risk

1. **Heavy Lifting Without Proper Technique**

   • Even outside of work, lifting heavy objects without using proper body mechanics can lead to hernias. This includes activities like moving furniture, carrying groceries, or lifting children.

2. **Repetitive Strain**

   • Activities that require repeated bending, twisting, or lifting can gradually weaken the abdominal muscles and increase the risk of hernia development.

3. **Prolonged Standing or Sitting**

   • Jobs that require long periods of standing or sitting can contribute to increased abdominal pressure, especially if combined with other risk factors like obesity or weak core muscles.

4. **Sudden Physical Exertion**

   • Sudden, intense physical effort, such as pushing a stalled car or lifting a heavy object unexpectedly, can cause a hernia by overwhelming the abdominal wall's capacity to contain internal organs and tissues.

Preventive Measures for High-Risk Occupations

1. **Ergonomic Training**

- Learning and consistently applying proper lifting techniques, such as lifting with the legs instead of the back, can significantly reduce the risk of hernias.

2. **Core Strengthening Exercises**

- Regular exercise to strengthen the core muscles helps provide better support for the abdominal wall, making it less prone to hernias.

3. **Use of Assistive Devices**

- In occupations involving heavy lifting, using tools like hoists, pulleys, or dollies can reduce the physical strain on the body.

4. **Taking Regular Breaks**

- Short breaks during long periods of standing or sitting can help alleviate the buildup of pressure in the abdominal area.

By recognizing the occupational hazards associated with hernias, individuals and employers can take proactive steps to minimize risk and protect workers from this common health issue. The next section will explore how medical conditions can also play a role in hernia development, adding another layer to our understanding of risk factors.

Medical Conditions and Hernias

Certain medical conditions can predispose individuals to hernias by weakening the abdominal wall or increasing intra-abdominal pressure. Chronic illnesses and disorders that involve persistent strain, tissue weakness, or increased abdominal pressure significantly contribute to hernia development. Let's explore the connection between specific medical conditions and hernias.

Chronic Illnesses and Their Connection to Hernias

1. Chronic Obstructive Pulmonary Disease (COPD)

• **Coughing:** One of the primary symptoms of COPD is chronic coughing. Persistent and forceful coughing increases intra-abdominal pressure, which can strain the abdominal wall, leading to the formation of hernias, particularly in the inguinal and umbilical regions.

• **General Weakness:** COPD can also lead to generalized muscle weakness, which affects the integrity of the abdominal wall, further increasing hernia risk.

2. Asthma

• Similar to COPD, asthma involves frequent coughing and difficulty breathing, which can cause repeated increases in intra-abdominal pressure, leading to hernias over time.

3. Chronic Constipation

• **Straining:** Regular straining during bowel movements due to constipation puts significant pressure on the abdominal wall, making it a common cause of hernias, especially inguinal and umbilical hernias.

• **Repeated Episodes:** Chronic constipation leads to repeated strain over months or years, gradually weakening the abdominal muscles and fascia.

4. Benign Prostatic Hyperplasia (BPH)

• **Difficulty Urinating:** Men with BPH often experience difficulty urinating, leading to frequent straining. This prolonged and repetitive pressure can cause or exacerbate inguinal hernias.

5. Cystic Fibrosis

• **Chronic Coughing:** Like COPD and asthma, cystic fibrosis involves chronic coughing, which increases the risk of hernia development due to the constant elevation of intra-abdominal pressure.

• **Digestive Issues:** The condition also affects the digestive system, contributing to constipation and further elevating the risk.

6. Obesity

• **Excess Weight:** Carrying excess weight puts continuous pressure on the abdominal wall, weakening it over time and making it more susceptible to hernias.

• **Fatigue and Weakness:** Obesity can also lead to overall muscle weakness, reducing the body's ability to support the internal organs properly.

7. Ascites

• **Fluid Accumulation:** Ascites, the accumulation of fluid in the abdominal cavity, increases intra-abdominal pressure, often leading to hernias, especially umbilical hernias.

• **Chronic Conditions:** Ascites is commonly associated with liver diseases like cirrhosis, which also weaken the body's overall strength and resilience.

8. Pregnancy

• **Abdominal Strain:** The growing uterus during pregnancy stretches and weakens the abdominal muscles, which can lead to hernias, particularly umbilical and incisional hernias.

• **Multiple Pregnancies:** Women with multiple pregnancies are at a higher risk due to the repeated stretching and strain on the abdominal wall.

9. Collagen Disorders

• **Weak Connective Tissue:** Disorders like Ehlers-Danlos syndrome and Marfan syndrome involve genetic defects in collagen, a vital component of connective tissue. These conditions inherently weaken the structural integrity of the abdominal wall, making hernias more likely.

10.   Diabetes

• **Delayed Healing:** Diabetes can impair the body's healing process, particularly after surgery or injury, increasing the risk of incisional hernias.

• **Tissue Quality:** Long-term diabetes can also degrade tissue quality, weakening the abdominal wall and making it more susceptible to hernias.

Managing Medical Conditions to Reduce Hernia Risk

1. **Proper Management of Chronic Illnesses**

   • Controlling chronic conditions like COPD, asthma, and constipation through medications and lifestyle changes can reduce the strain on the abdominal wall and decrease hernia risk.

2. **Weight Management**

   • Maintaining a healthy weight through diet and exercise can reduce the continuous pressure on the abdominal muscles, significantly lowering the likelihood of hernia development.

3. **Avoiding Straining**

   • For conditions like BPH and chronic constipation, medical treatments and dietary changes to ease straining can help prevent hernias.

4. **Regular Monitoring**

   • Individuals with chronic illnesses that increase hernia risk should undergo regular check-ups to monitor for early signs of hernia development.

By understanding the link between chronic illnesses and hernias, individuals can take proactive steps to manage their health and reduce the risk of hernias, enhancing their overall well-being. The next chapter will delve into the symptoms of hernias and how to recognize them early for prompt treatment.

Chapter 3: Symptoms and Diagnosis

Early Warning Signs

Recognizing the early warning signs of hernias is crucial for prompt diagnosis and treatment. While the symptoms can vary depending on the type of hernia, some common indicators can help identify the condition early. In this section, we'll discuss the typical symptoms associated with different types of hernias and highlight the importance of early detection.

Common Symptoms for Different Types of Hernias

1. **Inguinal Hernia (Groin Area)**

   • **Visible Bulge:** One of the most noticeable signs is a bulge in the groin area, which may become more prominent when standing, coughing, or lifting heavy objects.

   • **Pain or Discomfort:** Some people experience a dull ache or burning sensation in the groin, especially during physical activity or prolonged standing.

   • **Weakness or Pressure:** A feeling of weakness or pressure in the groin area can indicate the presence of an inguinal hernia.

2. **Femoral Hernia**

• **Bulge Near the Thigh:** Similar to inguinal hernias, femoral hernias create a bulge, but this one is located just below the groin in the upper thigh area.

• **Discomfort or Pain:** Pain may be felt in the groin or upper thigh, particularly when lifting or straining.

• **More Common in Women:** Femoral hernias are more frequently diagnosed in women, often due to the wider pelvis structure.

3. **Umbilical Hernia**

• **Bulge Near the Navel:** A soft bulge near the navel, which can increase in size when coughing, crying (in infants), or straining, is a typical symptom.

• **Pain or Tenderness:** Some may experience tenderness or discomfort around the bulge, especially when the hernia is large or under pressure.

4. **Hiatal Hernia**

• **Heartburn and Acid Reflux:** One of the most common symptoms is persistent heartburn or acid reflux, as the stomach pushes up through the diaphragm.

• **Difficulty Swallowing:** A hiatal hernia can cause difficulty swallowing (dysphagia), particularly if the hernia is large enough to compress the esophagus.

• **Chest Pain:** Some individuals experience chest pain or discomfort, which can be mistaken for heart problems.

5. **Incisional Hernia**

• **Bulge Near a Surgical Scar:** A noticeable bulge near the site of a previous surgical incision is a primary symptom of an incisional hernia.

• **Discomfort or Pain:** Pain around the bulge, particularly when straining or lifting, is common.

• **Changes Over Time:** The bulge may increase in size over time, especially if not properly managed.

Importance of Early Detection

Early detection of hernias can prevent complications such as incarceration (where the hernia gets stuck in the opening) or strangulation (where the blood supply to the herniated tissue is cut off), both of which can be medical emergencies. Recognizing the symptoms and seeking medical advice promptly can lead to more effective management, whether through lifestyle changes, supportive measures, or surgical intervention.

In the next section, we'll explore how hernias are diagnosed, including the tools and techniques healthcare providers use to confirm the presence and type of hernia.

Diagnostic Tools and Techniques

Diagnosing a hernia involves a combination of clinical examination and imaging techniques to confirm the presence and type of hernia. Understanding these diagnostic tools and knowing when to seek medical attention can help ensure timely and effective treatment. In this section, we'll discuss the methods healthcare providers use to diagnose hernias and the signs that indicate it's time to consult a doctor.

Imaging and Clinical Examination Methods

1. **Clinical Examination**

    • **Physical Examination:** The first step in diagnosing a hernia is often a thorough physical exam. The doctor will check for visible bulges, especially in the abdomen or groin area, and may ask the patient to cough, strain, or stand up to make the hernia more apparent.

    • **Palpation:** The healthcare provider will use their hands to feel the affected area, checking for tenderness, the presence of a bulge, and whether the hernia can be pushed back into place (reducibility).

2. **Imaging Techniques**

    • **Ultrasound:** This non-invasive imaging technique uses sound waves to create images of the internal structures, making it useful for diagnosing hernias, especially in children or when the hernia is not clearly visible.

    • **CT Scan (Computed Tomography):** A CT scan provides detailed cross-sectional images of the body, which can help identify the size, location, and contents of a hernia, as well as detect complications such as strangulation.

    • **MRI (Magnetic Resonance Imaging):** MRI is particularly useful for diagnosing less obvious hernias, such as those in the groin or abdominal wall, by offering high-resolution images of soft tissues.

- **X-Ray:** In cases of hiatal hernias or complications like bowel obstruction, a chest or abdominal X-ray might be used to assess the condition of the digestive tract.

3. **Endoscopy (For Hiatal Hernias)**

- **Upper Endoscopy (EGD):** This procedure involves inserting a thin, flexible tube with a camera down the throat to view the esophagus and stomach, helping to diagnose hiatal hernias and associated conditions like gastroesophageal reflux disease (GERD).

When to See a Doctor

Knowing when to seek medical attention is crucial for preventing complications and ensuring proper management of hernias. Here are some indicators that it's time to consult a doctor:

1. **Persistent or Worsening Symptoms**

- If you notice a bulge that doesn't go away or keeps getting larger, or if you experience persistent discomfort or pain, it's important to see a doctor for an evaluation.

2. **Pain or Discomfort During Daily Activities**

- Pain that interferes with daily activities, such as walking, lifting, or standing for long periods, warrants medical attention.

3. **Difficulty Swallowing or Breathing (Hiatal Hernias)**

- For hiatal hernias, symptoms like persistent heartburn, acid reflux, difficulty swallowing, or chest pain should prompt a visit to the doctor.

4. **Signs of Complications**

    • **Incarceration:** A hernia that cannot be pushed back in (reduced) may be incarcerated, which can lead to severe pain, nausea, vomiting, or constipation.

    • **Strangulation:** If the hernia becomes strangulated, cutting off blood supply to the tissue, symptoms like sudden severe pain, redness or discoloration of the bulge, and systemic symptoms like fever require immediate emergency care.

5. **Post-Surgical Concerns (Incisional Hernias)**

    • If you've had abdominal surgery and notice a bulge near the incision site or experience pain and tenderness in that area, it's essential to consult your surgeon or a healthcare provider.

By understanding the diagnostic methods and knowing when to seek medical advice, individuals can take proactive steps to manage their health. Early diagnosis of hernias can lead to better outcomes, reducing the risk of complications and improving the effectiveness of treatment.

Chapter 4: Prevention Strategies

Strengthening Core Muscles

Strengthening the core muscles is one of the most effective strategies for preventing hernias. The core provides structural support to the abdominal wall and helps maintain intra-abdominal pressure, reducing the likelihood of developing a hernia. By incorporating specific exercises into your routine, you can strengthen these muscles and protect your body from strain. In this section, we'll discuss the importance of core strength and provide a range of exercises designed to reduce hernia risk.

Why Core Strength Matters for Hernia Prevention

The core muscles—comprising the muscles of the abdomen, lower back, and pelvis—play a critical role in maintaining proper posture, supporting the spine, and providing stability to the body. When these muscles are weak, the abdominal wall is less capable of withstanding the pressure exerted during activities like lifting, bending, or even coughing. This can increase the risk of hernia development.

A strong core helps to:

•   **Support the abdominal wall**: A well-developed core provides a stable foundation that can better absorb and distribute pressure during physical activity.

• **Maintain intra-abdominal pressure**: When you lift, cough, or strain, your core muscles work to stabilize the abdominal cavity, reducing the risk of the internal organs pushing through weak spots in the abdominal wall.

• **Prevent strain on surrounding muscles**: Strengthening the core reduces unnecessary strain on the lower back and pelvic muscles, which are often involved in hernia formation.

Core Strengthening Exercises to Reduce Hernia Risk

1. **Planks**

   • **How to Do It:** Start in a push-up position with your elbows bent at 90 degrees. Keep your body in a straight line from head to heels, engaging your core throughout. Hold this position for 20-30 seconds and gradually increase as your strength improves.

   • **Benefits:** Planks engage the entire core, helping to build strength and stability in the abdominal muscles and lower back.

2. **Bridges**

   • **How to Do It:** Lie on your back with your knees bent and feet flat on the floor, hip-width apart. Slowly lift your hips toward the ceiling, squeezing your glutes and engaging your abdominal muscles. Hold for a few seconds at the top, then lower your hips back to the ground.

   • **Benefits:** Bridges strengthen the glutes, lower back, and abdominal muscles, helping to reinforce the support for the pelvis and abdominal cavity.

3. **Bird Dogs**

- **How to Do It:** Start on your hands and knees, with your wrists aligned under your shoulders and knees under your hips. Extend your right arm forward and your left leg backward, keeping your body in a straight line. Hold for a few seconds, then return to the starting position. Repeat on the opposite side.

- **Benefits:** Bird dogs improve core stability and balance while strengthening the lower back, abs, and glutes.

4. **Leg Raises**

- **How to Do It:** Lie on your back with your legs straight. Slowly raise your legs towards the ceiling while keeping your lower back pressed into the floor. Lower your legs back down without letting them touch the ground.

- **Benefits:** Leg raises target the lower abdominal muscles, which are crucial for stabilizing the pelvic and abdominal regions.

5. **Dead Bugs**

- **How to Do It:** Lie on your back with your arms extended straight above you and your knees bent at 90 degrees. Slowly lower your right arm and left leg toward the floor, keeping your lower back pressed into the ground. Return to the starting position and repeat on the opposite side.

- **Benefits:** Dead bugs activate the core and help build strength and control in the abdominal muscles, promoting better stability for the entire abdominal wall.

6. **Russian Twists**

- **How to Do It:** Sit on the floor with your knees bent and feet flat, leaning slightly back to engage your core. Hold a weight or medicine ball with both hands and twist your torso to the left, then to the right, while keeping your hips stable.

- **Benefits:** This exercise targets the obliques, which are important muscles for rotational stability and overall abdominal strength.

7. **Cat-Cow Stretch**

- **How to Do It:** Begin on all fours with your wrists under your shoulders and knees under your hips. Inhale as you arch your back, letting your belly drop toward the floor (Cow), then exhale as you round your back, tucking your chin to your chest (Cat).

- **Benefits:** This dynamic movement improves spinal mobility and flexibility, while also activating the core muscles.

Additional Tips for Preventing Hernias

1. **Proper Lifting Techniques**

- Always engage your core before lifting heavy objects. Use your legs, not your back, to lift. Avoid twisting while lifting and instead pivot your feet to turn.

2. **Weight Management**

- Maintaining a healthy weight reduces the strain on your abdominal muscles and the pressure on the hernia-prone areas.

3. **Avoiding Excessive Strain**

• Limit activities that involve excessive straining, such as prolonged coughing, sneezing, or lifting heavy loads. If you have conditions like chronic cough or constipation, managing these can reduce the risk of developing a hernia.

4. **Pelvic Floor Exercises**

• In addition to core exercises, strengthening the pelvic floor through exercises like Kegels can provide additional support to the abdominal region, particularly for women after childbirth.

By incorporating these exercises and lifestyle changes into your routine, you can significantly reduce the risk of developing a hernia. Strengthening the core not only helps with hernia prevention but also improves overall posture, stability, and functional strength, benefiting your entire body.

Proper Lifting Techniques

Lifting is an essential part of daily life, whether you're carrying groceries, lifting a child, or moving furniture. However, improper lifting techniques can significantly increase your risk of developing a hernia. The way you lift determines how much strain is placed on your abdominal muscles, pelvic floor, and spine. In this section, we will cover the fundamental principles of safe lifting and tips for incorporating these techniques into your daily routine to reduce the risk of injury and hernias.

Tips for Safe Lifting in Daily Life

1. **Engage Your Core Before Lifting**

• **Why:** Engaging your core muscles helps stabilize the abdomen and spine, providing support during the lifting motion.

• **How:** Before lifting, tighten your abdominal muscles as if you're preparing to take a punch. This engagement helps reduce unnecessary strain on the abdominal wall.

2. **Bend at the Knees, Not the Waist**

• **Why:** Bending at the waist places excessive strain on the lower back and abdominal muscles. Instead, bending at the knees ensures that your legs, which are stronger and more capable of bearing weight, do the heavy lifting.

• **How:** Stand with your feet shoulder-width apart. Bend at the knees (not at the waist) to lower your body toward the object, keeping your back straight and chest lifted. This position maintains proper spinal alignment.

3. **Keep the Object Close to Your Body**

• **Why:** The farther an object is from your body, the more force your abdominal and lower back muscles must generate to lift it. This increases the risk of injury or developing a hernia.

• **How:** As you lift, hold the object as close to your body as possible. This reduces the strain on your core muscles and spine. The closer the weight is to your center of gravity, the easier it is to lift safely.

4. **Use Your Legs to Lift, Not Your Back**

• **Why:** The legs are stronger muscles than the back, so they should be the primary source of power when lifting. Using your back to lift increases the risk of straining the muscles of the lower back and abdomen.

• **How:** As you lower yourself to lift, focus on pushing with your legs rather than bending forward with your back. Straighten your legs slowly to lift the object, maintaining a stable torso.

5. **Keep a Neutral Spine**

• **Why:** Maintaining a neutral spine (a straight, aligned back) during lifting reduces the risk of injury to the spine, abdominal muscles, and pelvic floor.

• **How:** Keep your back straight, shoulders pulled back, and chest lifted as you lift the object. Avoid rounding your back or twisting your torso while lifting.

6. **Avoid Twisting While Lifting**

• **Why:** Twisting your torso while lifting can put additional strain on your abdominal muscles and lower back, increasing the risk of hernias and other injuries.

• **How:** If you need to turn or change direction while lifting, move your feet first instead of twisting your back. Pivot your feet to change direction smoothly without twisting your spine.

7. **Don't Overexert Yourself**

• **Why:** Lifting too heavy an object can put excessive pressure on your abdominal wall and spine, increasing the risk of injury and hernia development.

• **How:** If an object feels too heavy or awkward to lift alone, ask for help or use assistive devices like a dolly or lifting straps to share the load.

8. **Take Breaks for Repetitive Lifting**

   • **Why:** Repetitive lifting, especially with poor technique, can lead to fatigue and strain on the muscles, increasing the risk of injury.

   • **How:** If you're lifting multiple objects or engaging in a prolonged activity (like moving boxes), take frequent breaks to rest and re-engage your core before lifting again.

9. **Plan Your Lifts**

   • **Why:** Lifting with forethought minimizes the need for awkward movements or unnecessary strain.

   • **How:** Before lifting, assess the size, weight, and position of the object. Plan the route you will take, and ensure that there are no obstacles in your path that might cause you to twist or lose your balance.

Additional Tips for Specific Scenarios

1. **Lifting Children or Pets**

   • When lifting small children or pets, bend at your knees, keep the child or pet close to your body, and use your legs to lift rather than your back. This ensures that the lift is safe for both your body and the child or pet.

2. **Lifting Large or Awkward Items (e.g., Furniture)**

   • For large or bulky objects, break the load down into smaller, more manageable parts if possible. If it is a one-person lift, ensure you have a clear path and use proper lifting equipment like furniture sliders or a hand truck.

3. **Lifting Objects from the Floor**

• When lifting something off the floor, keep your knees bent, maintain a straight back, and bend at the hips, not the waist. This will prevent unnecessary strain on the lower back and abdominal muscles.

By incorporating these safe lifting practices into your daily life, you can significantly reduce the risk of developing a hernia and protect your body from injury. Remember that lifting with proper form isn't just important for preventing hernias—it's essential for long-term spinal health and overall muscle function.

Dietary Considerations

Diet plays an essential role in supporting overall health, including the strength and integrity of the tissues in your abdominal wall, as well as aiding digestion and preventing unnecessary strain on your body. Proper nutrition can reduce the risk of developing a hernia, improve tissue healing after surgery, and support digestive function. In this section, we will explore foods that promote tissue health, support digestion, and help prevent conditions that may contribute to hernia formation.

Foods that Support Tissue Health

1. **Protein-Rich Foods**

• **Why:** Protein is the building block of tissues, including muscles, ligaments, and connective tissue. Adequate protein intake helps to maintain the strength and elasticity of the abdominal wall, making it more resilient to pressure and strain.

• **Sources:** Lean meats (chicken, turkey, lean beef), fish (salmon, tuna), eggs, tofu, legumes (beans, lentils), and dairy products (Greek yogurt, cottage cheese).

2. **Collagen-Boosting Foods**

• **Why:** Collagen is a major component of connective tissue, providing strength and structure. Collagen helps maintain the elasticity of the abdominal wall, which is vital for preventing hernias and improving recovery after surgery.

• **Sources:** Bone broth, chicken skin, fish skin, and collagen supplements. Additionally, foods that support collagen production include vitamin C-rich foods.

3. **Vitamin C-Rich Foods**

• **Why:** Vitamin C plays a critical role in collagen synthesis, which is essential for tissue repair and the health of connective tissues.

• **Sources:** Citrus fruits (oranges, lemons), bell peppers, strawberries, kiwi, tomatoes, and broccoli.

4. **Omega-3 Fatty Acids**

• **Why:** Omega-3 fatty acids have anti-inflammatory properties, which can help reduce chronic inflammation and support overall tissue repair.

• **Sources:** Fatty fish (salmon, mackerel, sardines), flaxseeds, chia seeds, walnuts, and omega-3-rich oils (like olive oil and flaxseed oil).

5. **Zinc-Rich Foods**

• **Why:** Zinc is crucial for tissue healing and immune function. It helps in collagen formation and wound healing, which can benefit those recovering from surgery or preventing hernia-related complications.

- **Sources:** Shellfish (oysters, crab), lean meats, beans, nuts, seeds, whole grains, and dairy products.

6. **Vitamin E**

- **Why:** Vitamin E is a powerful antioxidant that can help protect tissues from oxidative damage and promote healthy skin and connective tissue.

- **Sources:** Nuts, seeds, spinach, broccoli, and avocados.

Foods that Support Digestion

1. **Fiber-Rich Foods**

- **Why:** A high-fiber diet supports healthy digestion and prevents constipation, a common risk factor for developing a hernia, particularly inguinal and umbilical hernias. Straining during bowel movements increases intra-abdominal pressure, which can contribute to hernia formation.

- **Sources:** Whole grains (brown rice, quinoa, oats), fruits (apples, berries, pears), vegetables (leafy greens, carrots, broccoli), legumes (beans, lentils), and nuts.

2. **Hydrating Foods**

- **Why:** Staying hydrated is vital for digestive health. Dehydration can lead to constipation and difficulty passing stools, which in turn can increase the risk of developing a hernia.

- **Sources:** Water, herbal teas, and hydrating fruits and vegetables (cucumbers, watermelon, celery, oranges).

3. **Probiotic Foods**

• **Why:** Probiotics support a healthy gut microbiome, which is essential for optimal digestion and nutrient absorption. A balanced gut can help reduce bloating, gas, and other digestive issues that might contribute to abdominal pressure.

• **Sources:** Yogurt with live cultures, kefir, sauerkraut, kimchi, miso, and kombucha.

4. **Digestive Enzyme-Rich Foods**

• **Why:** Foods that contain natural digestive enzymes can support better digestion and reduce bloating or discomfort in the abdominal area, reducing strain on the abdominal wall.

• **Sources:** Pineapple (bromelain), papaya (papain), and fermented foods like sauerkraut and kimchi.

5. **Healthy Fats**

• **Why:** Healthy fats support cellular function, including the health of tissues in the abdominal region. They also promote satiety and help with the absorption of fat-soluble vitamins (A, D, E, K) that are essential for tissue repair.

• **Sources:** Avocados, olive oil, coconut oil, nuts, and seeds.

Foods to Avoid

1. **Processed Foods and Sugars**

• **Why:** Processed foods and excess sugar can increase inflammation and disrupt normal digestive function. Chronic inflammation can impair tissue repair and may contribute to the weakening of the abdominal wall over time.

• **Sources to Avoid:** Sugary drinks, sweets, pastries, and foods high in refined carbohydrates and artificial additives.

2. **Excessive Salt**

• **Why:** Too much salt can lead to water retention, bloating, and increased pressure in the abdominal cavity. This can exacerbate issues related to hernias or abdominal discomfort.

• **Sources to Avoid:** Fast food, canned foods, and processed meats.

3. **Caffeinated and Carbonated Beverages**

• **Why:** Caffeine and carbonated drinks can contribute to bloating and indigestion, both of which can increase abdominal pressure and strain the abdominal wall.

• **Sources to Avoid:** Soda, energy drinks, excessive coffee, and alcoholic beverages.

Sample Meal Plan for Hernia Prevention

Here is a sample meal plan that incorporates foods that support tissue health and digestion while avoiding those that may increase risk factors:

Breakfast:

• Oatmeal topped with chia seeds, walnuts, and berries

• A glass of water or herbal tea

Lunch:

•   Grilled chicken salad with leafy greens, bell peppers, avocado, and olive oil dressing

•   A whole grain roll or quinoa on the side

•   A glass of water

Snack:

•   Greek yogurt with a handful of pumpkin seeds and fresh fruit (like kiwi or strawberries)

Dinner:

•   Baked salmon with steamed broccoli and sweet potato

•   A side of sautéed spinach with garlic and olive oil

•   A glass of water

Evening Snack:

•   A small handful of almonds or a few slices of avocado with a sprinkle of sea salt

By incorporating these nutrient-dense foods into your daily meals, you can help support the strength of your abdominal tissues, improve digestion, and lower the risk of developing a hernia. A well-balanced diet is not only beneficial for hernia prevention but also for overall health and well-being.

Managing Chronic Conditions

Chronic conditions, particularly those that impact the digestive system, abdominal pressure, or overall muscle integrity, can exacerbate the risk of developing or worsening a hernia. Managing these conditions through proper medical care, lifestyle modifications, and dietary strategies can significantly reduce the risk of hernia complications and improve quality of life. In this section, we will discuss several chronic conditions that may contribute to hernias and provide actionable strategies for managing these conditions to minimize their impact.

Chronic Conditions That May Exacerbate Hernias

1. **Chronic Obstructive Pulmonary Disease (COPD)**

   • **How it Affects Hernias:** Chronic coughing is a hallmark symptom of COPD, and frequent coughing can increase intra-abdominal pressure, potentially causing or worsening a hernia, particularly a hiatal or inguinal hernia.

   • **Management Strategies:**

      • **Quit Smoking:** Smoking exacerbates COPD and impairs lung function, increasing the frequency and intensity of coughing. Quitting smoking can improve lung health and reduce the strain on your abdominal muscles.

      • **Cough Management:** Work with your doctor to manage chronic cough effectively. This may include medications (e.g., bronchodilators, corticosteroids) and pulmonary rehabilitation to strengthen respiratory muscles and reduce the urge to cough.

• **Breathing Exercises:** Incorporating deep breathing techniques can help reduce the frequency of coughing and support better lung function, which in turn helps control abdominal pressure.

2. **Constipation**

• **How it Affects Hernias:** Straining during bowel movements increases intra-abdominal pressure, putting excessive strain on the abdominal wall and increasing the likelihood of developing or exacerbating a hernia.

• **Management Strategies:**

• **Increase Fiber Intake:** A high-fiber diet (including whole grains, fruits, vegetables, and legumes) can help soften stools and promote regular bowel movements.

• **Stay Hydrated:** Drinking plenty of water helps keep stools soft and easier to pass, reducing the need to strain during bowel movements.

• **Regular Exercise:** Regular physical activity, including abdominal-strengthening exercises, helps maintain healthy digestion and prevents constipation.

• **Over-the-Counter Remedies:** Use stool softeners or mild laxatives only when necessary and under the guidance of your doctor to avoid worsening constipation over time.

3. **Obesity**

• **How it Affects Hernias:** Excess weight places added pressure on the abdominal wall, which can weaken tissues over time and contribute to the formation or worsening of hernias, particularly abdominal hernias like umbilical or incisional hernias.

• **Management Strategies:**

• **Healthy Weight Loss:** Aim for gradual weight loss through a balanced diet and regular physical activity. Reducing abdominal fat can alleviate pressure on the abdominal wall and improve overall health.

• **Focus on Core Strengthening:** In addition to weight loss, exercises that strengthen the core muscles (like planks, bridges, and leg raises) will help provide stability to the abdominal wall and reduce hernia risk.

• **Work with a Dietitian:** A registered dietitian can help you create a personalized eating plan that supports healthy weight loss while ensuring adequate nutrient intake for tissue repair and overall health.

4. **Gastroesophageal Reflux Disease (GERD)**

• **How it Affects Hernias:** GERD can contribute to the development of a hiatal hernia, a condition in which part of the stomach pushes through the diaphragm into the chest cavity. Acid reflux and heartburn may worsen due to the pressure from a hernia.

• **Management Strategies:**

- **Eat Smaller, More Frequent Meals:** Eating large meals can increase pressure on the stomach and worsen reflux symptoms. Try eating smaller meals more frequently throughout the day.

- **Avoid Trigger Foods:** Certain foods (like spicy foods, chocolate, caffeine, and alcohol) can irritate the stomach lining and worsen acid reflux. Identify and avoid your personal triggers.

- **Elevate the Head of Your Bed:** If you experience nighttime acid reflux, try elevating the head of your bed to reduce stomach acid from flowing into the esophagus while you sleep.

- **Medications:** Over-the-counter antacids, H2 blockers, and proton pump inhibitors can help control GERD symptoms and reduce the risk of developing a hiatal hernia. Consult your doctor for appropriate treatment.

5. **Cystic Fibrosis**

- **How it Affects Hernias:** Individuals with cystic fibrosis often experience chronic coughing, which can increase intra-abdominal pressure and contribute to hernia formation, especially in the abdominal area.

- **Management Strategies:**

- **Pulmonary Treatment:** Follow the prescribed regimen of medications and physical therapies to reduce coughing episodes. This may include bronchodilators, chest physiotherapy, and mucolytic agents to help clear mucus from the lungs.

- **Nutritional Support:** People with cystic fibrosis often require additional calories and specific nutrient supplementation. A nutritionist familiar with cystic fibrosis can help design an eating plan that promotes weight gain and maintains adequate muscle strength.

• **Regular Monitoring:** Regular medical checkups to monitor lung health and abdominal pressure are essential for early detection and prevention of complications like hernias.

6. Chronic Straining from Urinary Conditions (e.g., Benign Prostatic Hyperplasia)

• **How it Affects Hernias:** Conditions that require frequent straining during urination, such as benign prostatic hyperplasia (BPH), can increase pressure on the abdomen and lead to hernia formation or exacerbation.

• **Management Strategies:**

• **Manage Underlying Conditions:** Medications for BPH, such as alpha-blockers or 5-alpha-reductase inhibitors, can help reduce urinary symptoms and decrease the need to strain.

• **Timely Bathroom Visits:** Don't delay urination, and try to avoid holding your bladder for long periods, which can lead to straining.

• **Hydration and Dietary Modifications:** Maintain good hydration, as well as a diet rich in fiber, to promote regular bowel movements and reduce the likelihood of straining during urination or defecation.

General Strategies for Managing Chronic Conditions That Exacerbate Hernias

1. **Maintain Regular Medical Checkups**

   • Regular consultations with your healthcare provider are essential for managing chronic conditions. If you have a history of hernias or are at high risk, your doctor can help monitor your condition and recommend lifestyle changes or medications that reduce the risk of hernia formation.

2. **Maintain a Healthy Lifestyle**

   • Adopting a holistic approach to health, including a balanced diet, regular physical activity, and adequate sleep, can help reduce the impact of chronic conditions on hernia risk. These changes improve muscle strength, digestive function, and overall tissue health.

3. **Manage Stress Effectively**

   • Chronic stress can exacerbate conditions like GERD, constipation, and chronic coughing, all of which contribute to hernia formation. Practice stress management techniques like meditation, yoga, deep breathing exercises, or mindfulness to improve overall well-being.

By actively managing chronic conditions through medical interventions, lifestyle changes, and dietary strategies, you can significantly reduce the risk of developing or worsening a hernia. Proactively addressing underlying issues will not only protect your abdominal health but also improve your overall quality of life.

Chapter 5: Treatment Options

Treating a hernia can range from simple lifestyle modifications to more advanced medical interventions, depending on the severity of the condition. While surgery is often the most effective way to correct a hernia, there are several non-surgical treatment options that can help manage symptoms, prevent further complications, and improve quality of life. In this chapter, we will focus on non-surgical interventions, including lifestyle modifications and the use of support garments, as part of a comprehensive treatment plan.

Non-Surgical Interventions

Non-surgical treatments are often used in cases where the hernia is small, not causing significant symptoms, or if surgery is not immediately necessary due to other health factors. These treatments aim to manage the condition, alleviate discomfort, and reduce the risk of further complications. Below are the most common non-surgical approaches:

Lifestyle Modifications

1. **Dietary Changes**

   - **Why It Helps:** A balanced, anti-inflammatory diet can help reduce the strain on your abdomen, support tissue health, and prevent conditions (like constipation or acid reflux) that exacerbate hernias.

- **Key Dietary Modifications:**

    - **Increase Fiber Intake:** As mentioned earlier, a fiber-rich diet can prevent constipation, which often leads to straining and increased intra-abdominal pressure, contributing to the formation of hernias. Fiber sources include fruits, vegetables, whole grains, and legumes.

    - **Avoid Trigger Foods:** For individuals with a hiatal hernia, avoiding spicy foods, alcohol, caffeine, and fatty meals can reduce symptoms of acid reflux and prevent further damage to the esophagus.

    - **Hydrate Properly:** Staying hydrated is crucial for maintaining healthy digestion and preventing constipation, which could worsen hernia symptoms.

2. **Weight Management**

- **Why It Helps:** Excess weight puts additional pressure on the abdominal wall, increasing the risk of hernia development or worsening an existing hernia.

- **How to Achieve It:**

    - **Balanced Diet:** Focus on a diet rich in whole foods like lean proteins, vegetables, and whole grains to promote healthy, sustainable weight loss.

    - **Exercise:** Incorporate moderate aerobic exercises (e.g., walking, swimming) and strength training (focusing on core muscles) to support weight loss while strengthening the abdominal muscles.

3. **Avoiding Straining and Heavy Lifting**

• **Why It Helps:** Activities that increase intra-abdominal pressure, such as heavy lifting, straining during bowel movements, or even intense coughing, can aggravate a hernia or increase the risk of a hernia becoming more pronounced.

• **Strategies:**

• **Lift with Proper Form:** Always bend at the knees and not at the waist when lifting heavy objects. Avoid twisting motions and be mindful of your posture.

• **Use Assistance:** When lifting heavy or bulky objects, consider using mechanical aids or asking for help to reduce strain.

• **Avoid Straining:** Regular bowel movements are essential, and strategies like increasing fiber intake, staying hydrated, and exercising can help prevent constipation and reduce the need for straining.

4. **Quit Smoking**

• **Why It Helps:** Smoking weakens connective tissue, impairing the healing process and increasing the risk of hernia formation. Additionally, smoking can lead to chronic coughing, which increases intra-abdominal pressure and aggravates hernia symptoms.

• **How to Achieve It:**

• **Smoking Cessation Programs:** Consider joining a smoking cessation program, using nicotine replacement therapy (NRT), or seeking support from a healthcare provider to help you quit.

• **Mindfulness and Stress Reduction:** Some people find that mindfulness practices and stress reduction techniques help them manage cravings and stay smoke-free.

Support Garments

Support garments are a non-invasive treatment option that can help manage symptoms of a hernia by providing external support to the abdominal wall. They are particularly useful for individuals who cannot undergo surgery immediately or are managing a hernia conservatively.

1. **Abdominal Binders**

• **What They Are:** Abdominal binders are elastic garments that wrap around the abdomen, providing support to the abdominal muscles and preventing the hernia from bulging further.

• **How They Help:**

• **Pressure Distribution:** They distribute pressure across the abdominal wall, reducing strain on the hernia site and preventing it from becoming larger or more painful.

• **Symptom Relief:** They can provide relief from pain or discomfort, especially during physical activity or when standing for extended periods.

• **Post-Surgery Use:** Abdominal binders are also used post-surgery to support the healing process and reduce swelling.

2. **Hernia Belts**

- **What They Are:** Hernia belts are similar to abdominal binders but are designed specifically for the type of hernia the individual has. For example, an inguinal hernia belt will be designed to apply pressure to the groin area, while an umbilical hernia belt targets the abdomen.

- **How They Help:**

    - **Localized Support:** These belts provide targeted compression on the hernia site, helping to keep the hernia from protruding or becoming more pronounced.

    - **Pain Relief:** They help alleviate the discomfort associated with hernias by reducing the pressure on the affected area.

    - **Activity-Specific Garments:** For individuals with an active lifestyle, these belts can provide added stability during exercise or heavy lifting.

3. **Trusses for Inguinal Hernias**

- **What They Are:** Trusses are devices designed specifically for inguinal hernias. They consist of a pad or cushion that is held in place with an adjustable strap around the waist or groin.

- **How They Help:**

    - **Pressure Relief:** The truss applies gentle pressure to the hernia site to keep the hernia from bulging out. It can be worn during physical activities to provide additional support.

•   **Comfortable Use:** Many modern trusses are designed to be worn discreetly under clothing, making them suitable for daily wear.

4. **Elastic Compression Garments**

• **What They Are:** These garments include compression shorts, underwear, or elastic belts that gently compress the abdominal area.

• **How They Help:**

•   **General Support:** These garments provide light compression to support the abdominal wall and reduce strain on the hernia, offering relief from mild discomfort.

•   **Prevention:** For those at risk of developing a hernia, elastic compression garments can provide preventive support during physical activity or lifting.

When to Seek Medical Advice

While lifestyle modifications and support garments can provide relief from mild hernia symptoms, it is essential to know when medical intervention is necessary. You should seek medical attention if:

•   The hernia becomes significantly painful or tender to the touch.

•   The hernia is rapidly increasing in size.

•   You experience nausea, vomiting, or difficulty passing stools.

•   The hernia becomes irreducible (it cannot be pushed back into place).

• You develop signs of complications, such as bowel obstruction or strangulation.

Summary

Non-surgical treatments for hernias can help manage symptoms, prevent the condition from worsening, and improve overall quality of life. By adopting lifestyle modifications, such as proper diet, weight management, and avoiding heavy lifting, you can reduce the strain on your abdominal muscles. Support garments like abdominal binders, hernia belts, and trusses provide external support and alleviate discomfort, particularly during physical activities. However, it is essential to remain vigilant about your symptoms and seek medical advice when necessary.

Surgical Treatments

While non-surgical interventions can help manage hernia symptoms and prevent further complications, surgery remains the definitive solution for many types of hernias, particularly when the hernia is causing pain, growing in size, or posing a risk of strangulation or other serious complications. Surgical treatment for hernias is generally safe and highly effective, with various approaches depending on the type of hernia, its severity, and the patient's overall health. In this section, we will explore different surgical approaches for hernia repair and examine the latest innovations in hernia surgery.

Different Surgical Approaches

1. **Open Hernia Repair (Traditional Surgery)**

• **What It Is:** In open hernia repair, the surgeon makes a single incision near the hernia site to access and repair the hernia. The protruding tissue (such as part of the intestine or abdominal fat) is pushed back into the abdomen, and the weakened area of the abdominal wall is reinforced with sutures or mesh.

• **When It's Used:** This method is typically used for larger hernias or when the hernia is located in a position that makes laparoscopic surgery difficult. It may also be the best option for patients with complex hernias or those with a history of previous abdominal surgeries.

• **Advantages:**

• Direct access to the hernia site allows for precise repair, particularly in complicated cases.

• Proven long-term effectiveness for preventing recurrence.

• **Disadvantages:**

• Larger incision means a longer recovery time and increased risk of infection.

• Hospital stay is typically longer than with laparoscopic surgery.

• Postoperative discomfort can be more significant.

2. **Laparoscopic Hernia Repair (Minimally Invasive Surgery)**

• **What It Is:** Laparoscopic surgery, also known as minimally invasive surgery, involves several small incisions (usually 3-4) through which the surgeon inserts a camera (laparoscope) and specialized surgical instruments to repair the hernia. The hernia is repaired using a mesh implant that strengthens the abdominal wall.

• **When It's Used:** Laparoscopic surgery is commonly used for inguinal hernias, especially in younger, healthier patients, and in cases where a quick recovery is desired.

• **Advantages:**

    • Smaller incisions mean less postoperative pain and faster recovery times.

    • Shorter hospital stays, often with the possibility of going home the same day.

    • Reduced risk of infection compared to open surgery.

    • Less visible scarring.

• **Disadvantages:**

    • It requires specialized equipment and a highly skilled surgeon.

    • There may be longer operating times compared to open surgery.

    • The approach may not be suitable for large or complicated hernias.

3. **Robotic Hernia Repair**

• **What It Is:** Robotic-assisted surgery is a variation of laparoscopic surgery in which the surgeon controls a robotic system to perform the procedure with enhanced precision. The surgeon uses a console to manipulate robotic arms equipped with small instruments and a high-definition camera.

• **When It's Used:** Robotic hernia repair is used in complex cases or when precision and dexterity are critical. It is increasingly popular for hernias in challenging anatomical areas or in patients with recurrent hernias.

• **Advantages:**

   • Greater precision and flexibility in the repair, particularly for difficult-to-reach hernias.

   • 3D visualization for better clarity and accuracy.

   • Smaller incisions, leading to faster recovery and less pain.

   • Reduced risk of complications like mesh migration or recurrence.

• **Disadvantages:**

   • Requires a highly trained surgeon and specialized robotic equipment.

   • The procedure may be more expensive due to the cost of robotic equipment.

   • The surgeon must be proficient in robotic techniques.

4. **Hernia Repair with Mesh**

• **What It Is:** Mesh is often used in both open and laparoscopic surgeries to reinforce the abdominal wall after the hernia has been reduced. The mesh acts as a "patch" that strengthens the area, reducing the risk of the hernia returning.

• **When It's Used:** Mesh is the standard in most hernia repairs, as it significantly reduces the risk of recurrence, particularly in large or complex hernias.

• **Advantages:**

    • Reduces the likelihood of the hernia returning.

    • Mesh provides a strong, flexible reinforcement for the abdominal wall.

    • Fewer complications and better long-term outcomes compared to non-mesh repairs.

• **Disadvantages:**

    • There is a small risk of mesh complications, including infection, migration, or adhesion to surrounding tissue.

    • Some patients may have allergic reactions or sensitivities to the material.

5. **Tension-Free Repair**

• **What It Is:** In tension-free repair, the surgeon uses mesh to reinforce the abdominal wall without pulling the surrounding tissue tight. This reduces the risk of tension-related complications, such as chronic pain or recurrence.

• **When It's Used:** This technique is particularly beneficial for hernias that may be prone to recurrence due to tension in the repaired area.

• **Advantages:**

- Reduces the risk of recurrence by preventing tension on the tissue.

- Faster recovery compared to traditional tension repairs.

- Less postoperative pain.

- **Disadvantages:**

  - Requires careful placement and suturing of the mesh to ensure proper support.

  - The long-term durability of tension-free repairs is still being studied.

Innovations in Hernia Surgery

1. **Enhanced Recovery After Surgery (ERAS) Protocols**

- **What It Is:** ERAS protocols are evidence-based practices designed to improve recovery after surgery. They include strategies to reduce stress, optimize pain management, and accelerate healing. For hernia surgery, ERAS may involve the use of non-opioid pain medications, early mobilization, and nutritional support.

- **Benefits:**

  - Faster recovery with reduced pain and discomfort.

  - Shorter hospital stays and reduced risk of complications.

  - Better overall patient outcomes.

2. **Bioabsorbable Mesh**

- **What It Is:** Traditional mesh implants used in hernia repairs are made from synthetic materials that can remain in the body for life. Bioabsorbable mesh is a newer innovation designed to be gradually absorbed by the body after a certain period.

- **Benefits:**

  - Reduces the long-term risk of complications related to permanent mesh, such as migration or infection.

  - Ideal for patients with certain health conditions, such as those who may need subsequent surgeries in the abdominal area.

  - Allows natural tissue healing while providing temporary support.

- **Challenges:**

  - More research is needed to determine the long-term outcomes and effectiveness of bioabsorbable mesh.

  - It may not be suitable for all types of hernias.

3. **Minimal Access Surgery (MAS) for Complex Hernias**

- **What It Is:** Minimal access surgery techniques are used for more complex or recurrent hernias, where traditional laparoscopic methods may not suffice. These techniques involve advanced technology, including robotic assistance or endoscopic instruments, to access difficult-to-reach hernia sites with minimal disruption to surrounding tissues.

- **Benefits:**

•   Provides a less invasive option for patients with complex or recurrent hernias.

•   Reduces the risk of complications, such as infection or damage to surrounding organs.

•   Faster recovery compared to open surgery.

• **Challenges:**

•   Requires highly skilled surgeons with specialized training.

•   Not universally available in all healthcare settings.

4. **Patient-Specific Hernia Mesh Design**

• **What It Is:** Advances in 3D printing and personalized medicine have allowed for the development of custom mesh implants that are specifically designed for each patient based on their unique anatomy and hernia characteristics.

• **Benefits:**

•   Custom mesh can provide better support and reduce the risk of complications, such as mesh migration or rejection.

•   Tailored to the specific needs of the patient, potentially improving long-term outcomes and reducing recurrence.

• **Challenges:**

•   Still in early stages of widespread adoption, with more research needed on its long-term efficacy.

- Custom mesh is more expensive compared to standard mesh implants.

Surgical treatment remains the most effective option for many hernias, particularly when non-surgical methods are insufficient. Open hernia repair, laparoscopic surgery, robotic-assisted surgery, and tension-free repair are all widely used approaches, each offering unique advantages and disadvantages depending on the patient's specific condition. Innovations like bioabsorbable mesh, robotic surgery, and patient-specific mesh are helping to advance hernia treatment, offering more personalized, effective, and minimally invasive options for patients. If surgery is recommended for your hernia, discuss the various surgical approaches with your surgeon to determine the best option for you.

Chapter 6: Post-Treatment Recovery

Undergoing hernia surgery can mark a significant turning point in your journey toward relief from hernia-related pain and discomfort. However, recovery is just as important as the surgery itself. Proper post-surgery care ensures that the repair site heals optimally, reduces the risk of complications, and helps you return to your daily activities as quickly and safely as possible.

Post-Surgery Care

Recovering from hernia surgery can vary depending on the type of surgery you had, your overall health, and how well you follow post-operative instructions. Most people are able to go home the same day after minimally invasive or laparoscopic hernia surgery, though some may require an overnight stay after open surgery, particularly for more complex cases. In either case, it's important to understand what to expect during your recovery and how to manage any discomfort or potential complications.

What to Expect After Surgery

1. **Initial Pain and Discomfort**

   • **Pain Management:** It's common to experience some pain or discomfort at the surgery site in the first few days following hernia surgery. This can include soreness, tightness, and mild swelling. The pain usually subsides as the healing process progresses, and your doctor will prescribe or recommend pain medication to help you manage discomfort.

• **Duration of Pain:** Pain levels typically peak within the first 48 hours and gradually improve. Most people can return to over-the-counter pain relievers, such as acetaminophen or ibuprofen, within a few days. Stronger pain medication may be prescribed if necessary for the first few days.

• **Rest and Relaxation:** Adequate rest is crucial in the initial stages of recovery. While it's important to avoid strenuous activities, gentle movement is encouraged to promote circulation and prevent complications like blood clots.

2. **Swelling and Bruising**

• **What It Is:** Mild swelling and bruising around the incision site are common and generally resolve within a few weeks. This is a normal part of the body's healing response.

• **What to Do:** You can apply ice packs to the affected area for 15-20 minutes at a time during the first 48 hours to reduce swelling and discomfort. Make sure to wrap the ice in a cloth to avoid direct contact with the skin.

3. **Bandages and Wound Care**

• **Incision Site:** Depending on the type of surgery you had, you may have one or several small incisions that require care. If your surgeon used stitches that dissolve on their own, you won't need to have them removed. For non-dissolvable stitches, a follow-up visit may be required to remove them.

• **Cleaning the Area:** Keep the incision clean and dry to prevent infection. Your surgeon will give you instructions on when and how to shower after surgery. If you notice any signs of infection (redness, warmth, drainage, or fever), contact your doctor immediately.

• **Dressing Changes:** You may be instructed to change the bandage on your incision site daily, but it's important to follow your surgeon's advice regarding when to do so. Keep the area covered as recommended until your follow-up visit.

4. **Dietary Adjustments**

• **Post-Surgery Diet:** You may not feel hungry immediately after surgery due to anesthesia or medications. Start with small amounts of light, bland foods like broth, crackers, and toast. Gradually introduce a more regular diet as you regain your appetite.

• **Constipation Prevention:** Pain medications, reduced activity levels, and anesthesia can sometimes cause constipation. Drink plenty of fluids, increase fiber intake (fruits, vegetables, whole grains), and stay active (as directed by your doctor) to prevent constipation. Your doctor may also recommend a stool softener if necessary.

5. **Physical Activity and Mobility**

• **Getting Moving:** After surgery, you'll be encouraged to walk around within the first 24 hours to prevent complications like blood clots and promote circulation. Start with short, gentle walks and gradually increase your activity level as you feel able.

• **Lifting Restrictions:** One of the most important aspects of post-surgery care is avoiding lifting heavy objects. For the first few weeks, avoid lifting anything heavier than 10 pounds. Your doctor will provide specific lifting guidelines based on your individual situation. Lifting can strain the surgical site and impede healing.

• **Driving and Work:** If you had laparoscopic surgery, you may be able to return to work and driving within 1-2 weeks, provided your pain is manageable and you can move comfortably. For more extensive open surgery, you may need to take 4-6 weeks off work, particularly if your job requires heavy lifting or strenuous activity.

Tips for a Smooth Recovery

1. **Follow Your Doctor's Instructions**

• **Why It's Important:** Your surgeon will provide detailed instructions tailored to your specific surgery and recovery needs. Follow these instructions carefully to reduce the risk of complications and ensure a smooth recovery. These instructions may include guidelines on medication, activity levels, and wound care.

• **Keep Follow-Up Appointments:** It's essential to attend follow-up visits with your surgeon to ensure proper healing. These appointments allow your doctor to assess the surgical site, remove any stitches if necessary, and address any concerns you may have.

2. **Manage Pain Effectively**

• **Pain Relief Strategies:** While some discomfort is to be expected after surgery, it's important to manage pain effectively so you can rest and heal. Use prescribed pain medications as directed and supplement with over-the-counter options like ibuprofen or acetaminophen if advised by your doctor.

• **Natural Pain Relief:** Gentle activities like walking or applying warm compresses may also help reduce pain. Focus on relaxation techniques, such as deep breathing exercises, to manage any anxiety or stress related to the recovery process.

3. **Avoid Straining or Excessive Movement**

• **Strain-Free Recovery:** One of the most important aspects of post-surgery care is avoiding activities that could strain the repaired area. Be mindful of how you move, and avoid bending, twisting, or lifting heavy objects. These actions can put pressure on the abdominal wall and interfere with the healing process.

• **Gradual Return to Activity:** While it's tempting to return to your regular routine, it's crucial to give your body time to heal. Gradually increase your activity level based on your surgeon's recommendations, and avoid returning to strenuous activities like heavy lifting, running, or intense exercise until you have fully healed.

4. **Support Your Immune System**

• **Nutrition for Healing:** Eating a well-balanced diet rich in nutrients like vitamins C and D, zinc, and protein can help promote tissue repair and support the immune system during the healing process. Focus on lean proteins (chicken, fish, legumes), fruits, vegetables, and whole grains.

• **Hydration:** Drink plenty of water throughout the recovery process to keep your body hydrated and support proper digestion. Dehydration can slow down recovery and increase the risk of complications, such as constipation.

5. **Stay in Communication with Your Healthcare Provider**

• **Monitor Symptoms:** It's essential to stay in touch with your healthcare provider, especially if you notice any signs of complications, such as excessive swelling, fever, redness or drainage at the incision site, or worsening pain. Early detection of complications can prevent more serious issues from developing.

• **Ask Questions:** Don't hesitate to reach out to your doctor with any questions or concerns you have. Whether it's about managing pain, dietary changes, or returning to physical activities, clear communication is key to ensuring a smooth recovery.

Post-treatment recovery after hernia surgery is a gradual process that requires attention to self-care, proper pain management, and patience.
By following your doctor's instructions, managing your pain effectively, and avoiding strain on the surgical site, you can ensure a smooth recovery and minimize the risk of complications. Adequate rest, proper nutrition, and gentle physical activity will help your body heal. Remember, recovery times vary depending on the type of surgery, so it's important to listen to your body and gradually return to your daily routine when you're ready.

Long-Term Management

Once your hernia surgery is behind you, the focus shifts to maintaining your health and preventing the recurrence of a hernia. While surgery can effectively resolve a hernia in the short term, the true success of the procedure is determined by how well you manage your recovery and lifestyle moving forward. Long-term management involves making conscious choices that support the integrity of your abdominal wall, preventing unnecessary strain, and ensuring you stay on top of your health with regular follow-up care.

Avoiding Recurrence

A key concern after any hernia surgery is the possibility of recurrence, which can happen if the underlying causes or risk factors are not properly managed. The good news is that with a few proactive steps, you can significantly reduce the chances of your hernia returning.

1. **Strengthen Core Muscles**

   • **Why It's Important:** Your abdominal muscles and the connective tissue around your abdomen play a crucial role in preventing the development of a hernia. A strong core provides better support to the abdominal wall and reduces the likelihood of future hernias.

   • **How to Strengthen:** Focus on gentle, low-impact exercises that target your core muscles. These can include activities such as pelvic tilts, abdominal bracing, and light pilates or yoga. Avoid heavy weightlifting or exercises that strain the abdominal region, particularly in the early stages of recovery.

• **Consistency is Key:** Strengthening your core should become a part of your long-term routine. Incorporating these exercises into your daily or weekly workouts can help maintain abdominal muscle strength and stability over time.

2. **Adopt Safe Lifting Practices**

• **Why It's Important:** Lifting heavy objects improperly puts significant strain on the abdominal wall, which can lead to recurrence, particularly in individuals with a history of hernias.

• **How to Lift Safely:** Always bend at the knees rather than the waist when lifting. This minimizes the strain on your lower back and abdomen. If something feels too heavy, ask for help or use a lifting aid.

• **Avoiding Sudden Movements:** Try not to make sudden or jerky movements when lifting, as these can place additional stress on the surgical site and surrounding tissues.

3. **Maintain a Healthy Weight**

• **Why It's Important:** Being overweight or obese increases the pressure on the abdominal wall, which can lead to the formation of new hernias or the recurrence of an existing one. Maintaining a healthy weight reduces this strain.

• **How to Maintain Weight:** Focus on a balanced diet that is rich in nutrients and low in processed foods. Regular physical activity, even in moderate amounts, can help manage weight effectively without overloading the abdominal muscles.

4. **Avoid Chronic Coughing or Straining**

• **Why It's Important:** Chronic coughing or excessive straining, such as from constipation, can create constant pressure on the abdominal wall and increase the likelihood of developing a hernia.

• **Managing a Chronic Cough:** If you have persistent coughing due to allergies, asthma, or a respiratory illness, work with your doctor to manage the underlying cause. Quitting smoking, if applicable, can also help improve lung health and reduce coughing.

• **Preventing Constipation:** Follow a fiber-rich diet, stay hydrated, and exercise regularly to maintain healthy bowel movements. If necessary, consult your healthcare provider for a stool softener or other interventions to avoid straining during bowel movements.

5. **Avoid Heavy Lifting for Several Weeks to Months Post-Surgery**

• **Why It's Important:** After surgery, it's crucial to give your abdominal muscles time to fully heal and regain their strength. Lifting heavy objects or engaging in intense physical activity too soon can compromise the healing process and contribute to a recurrence.

• **How Long to Wait:** Your doctor will provide specific guidelines about when you can safely return to lifting heavy objects. In general, you should avoid heavy lifting for at least 6 weeks post-surgery, depending on the type of surgery and your individual healing progress.

Importance of Follow-Up Care

Regular follow-up care after hernia surgery is vital not just for checking the initial surgical site, but also for monitoring long-term health and preventing complications. Your healthcare provider will schedule several follow-up appointments in the months following your surgery to ensure everything is healing as expected and to catch any potential issues early.

1. **Scheduled Check-Ups**

   • **Why They're Important:** Follow-up appointments allow your doctor to evaluate the surgical site, check for signs of infection, and monitor the healing progress. These appointments can also provide an opportunity for you to ask any questions or discuss concerns about your recovery.

   • **When to Schedule:** Your doctor will likely schedule your first follow-up appointment within a week or two after surgery. Additional check-ups may be scheduled at 1, 3, and 6 months post-surgery, depending on the nature of your surgery and recovery.

2. **Assessing for Recurrence**

   • **Why It's Important:** Even after successful surgery, there is always a risk of recurrence, particularly in individuals with a history of hernias or those who engage in activities that put pressure on the abdominal wall. Regular follow-up care provides an opportunity for early detection of any potential recurrence.

   • **What to Watch For:** If you experience new symptoms such as bulging, pain, or a feeling of pressure in the abdomen, contact your healthcare provider immediately. These could be signs that the hernia is returning.

3. **Managing Long-Term Health Conditions**

• **Why It's Important:** Certain medical conditions, such as obesity, diabetes, and chronic lung diseases, can increase the risk of hernia recurrence. Maintaining good control of these conditions is critical for your long-term health and hernia prevention.

• **How to Manage:** Work closely with your healthcare provider to monitor and manage any chronic conditions. This might include adjusting your diet, taking medications as prescribed, or getting regular exercise. Managing your overall health can significantly reduce the chances of a hernia reoccurring.

4. **Nutritional Guidance**

• **Why It's Important:** Proper nutrition plays an important role in healing and maintaining abdominal health. A diet rich in vitamins, minerals, and proteins supports tissue repair and strengthens your core muscles.

• **What to Focus On:** Ensure you're consuming enough fiber to support digestion and avoid constipation, which can place strain on the abdominal wall. Additionally, protein-rich foods like lean meats, legumes, and nuts help promote tissue regeneration and muscle strength.

5. **Psychological Support**

• **Why It's Important:** Undergoing surgery and managing a hernia can be mentally taxing, particularly if you experience setbacks or complications during recovery. Psychological support, whether through counseling, support groups, or simply talking with friends and family, can be crucial in your long-term recovery.

• **How to Seek Help:** If you're feeling anxious or depressed about your recovery or the possibility of recurrence, don't hesitate to reach out for support. A counselor, therapist, or support group can provide helpful tools for managing stress and coping with your emotional health during recovery.

Chapter 7: Special Considerations

While hernias are commonly associated with adults, they can also affect children, often requiring different management strategies due to their unique anatomical and developmental needs. Pediatric hernias tend to have distinct characteristics from those seen in adults, and understanding these differences is crucial for providing the best care for younger patients. This chapter will focus on hernias in children, shedding light on the causes, symptoms, and treatment options specifically for this population.

Hernias in Children

Hernias in children can occur for a variety of reasons, some of which are related to birth defects or developmental abnormalities. While adult hernias often develop due to lifestyle factors like heavy lifting or chronic pressure on the abdomen, pediatric hernias are usually congenital or related to early-life conditions. The two most common types of hernias in children are **inguinal hernias** and **umbilical hernias**, though other types, such as diaphragmatic or hiatal hernias, can also occur.

Unique Aspects of Pediatric Hernias

1. **Congenital vs. Acquired Hernias**

• **Congenital Hernias:** Many hernias in children are present at birth (congenital), meaning they develop during fetal development. The most common congenital hernias are **inguinal hernias** (affecting the groin area) and **umbilical hernias** (around the belly button). These hernias occur because of incomplete closure of certain openings in the abdominal wall or the passageways that were supposed to close before birth.

• **Acquired Hernias:** While less common, acquired hernias can develop in children due to factors like a chronic cough, constipation, or a sudden increase in abdominal pressure. However, these tend to be less frequent than congenital hernias.

2. **Inguinal Hernias in Children**

• **What It Is:** Inguinal hernias occur when part of the intestine or abdominal tissue bulges through a weak spot or opening in the groin. This is more common in boys, particularly those born prematurely.

• **Why It Happens:** The inguinal canal, which carries the spermatic cord in boys or round ligament in girls, is supposed to close after birth. If this closure doesn't occur fully, a hernia can develop.

• **Symptoms:** In children, inguinal hernias may appear as a small bulge in the groin, which may become more pronounced when the child cries or strains. In some cases, the hernia is visible only when the child is active, like when they cough or laugh.

• **Treatment:** Surgery is the primary treatment for inguinal hernias in children. Since these hernias are typically congenital, the condition will not resolve on its own and usually requires a pediatric surgeon to repair the opening in the abdominal wall.

3. **Umbilical Hernias in Children**

• **What It Is:** Umbilical hernias occur when a small portion of the intestine or abdominal tissue pushes through the abdominal wall near the belly button. This type of hernia is more common in infants.

• **Why It Happens:** During fetal development, the umbilical cord passes through an opening in the abdominal muscles. In most cases, this opening closes shortly after birth. However, in some children, the muscles around the belly button do not fully close, leaving a small hole where a hernia can form.

• **Symptoms:** An umbilical hernia is often easy to spot as a bulge at the belly button, particularly when the child is crying or straining. In some cases, the bulge is present at birth and may become more noticeable during the first few months of life.

• **Treatment:** Many umbilical hernias in infants close on their own by the age of 1-2 years. However, if the hernia persists or is causing discomfort, a pediatric surgeon may recommend surgical intervention to repair the hernia and close the opening.

4. **Diaphragmatic Hernias in Children**

• **What It Is:** A diaphragmatic hernia occurs when a portion of the intestines or organs pushes through the diaphragm, the muscle that separates the chest cavity from the abdomen. This type of hernia is less common but can be more serious because it affects the organs in the chest.

- **Why It Happens:** Diaphragmatic hernias are often congenital and result from a defect in the diaphragm that allows abdominal organs to move into the chest. These hernias can cause significant breathing and feeding difficulties in newborns.

- **Symptoms:** Symptoms in infants can include difficulty breathing, rapid breathing, and a blue tint to the skin (cyanosis), as the lungs are compressed by the abdominal organs.

- **Treatment:** Diaphragmatic hernias require immediate medical attention, and surgery is typically performed shortly after birth to move the organs back into the abdomen and repair the defect in the diaphragm.

5. **Hiatal Hernias in Children**

- **What It Is:** A hiatal hernia occurs when part of the stomach bulges up into the chest through the diaphragm. While more common in adults, especially older adults, hiatal hernias can also occur in children.

- **Why It Happens:** This hernia type occurs when the opening in the diaphragm (called the hiatus) is too large, allowing the stomach to push up into the chest. This is usually due to congenital defects but can also occur after traumatic injury.

- **Symptoms:** Hiatal hernias in children can cause symptoms such as difficulty swallowing, chest pain, and heartburn. In more severe cases, the hernia can cause vomiting and problems with digestion.

- **Treatment:** In many cases, hiatal hernias are managed with medication to reduce stomach acid and ease discomfort. However, surgery may be necessary in severe cases or if the hernia causes significant complications.

6. Incarcerated or Strangulated Hernias in Children

• **What It Is:** In some cases, the hernia may become trapped (incarcerated) or cut off from its blood supply (strangulated), which can lead to more serious complications, such as tissue death or infection.

• **Why It Happens:** If part of the intestine or abdominal tissue becomes stuck in the hernia, it can lead to a condition where the hernia cannot be pushed back into place, causing pain, swelling, and potential damage to the affected tissue.

• **Symptoms:** Symptoms of an incarcerated or strangulated hernia can include severe pain, redness or discoloration at the hernia site, vomiting, and a noticeable change in the child's behavior (e.g., excessive crying or lethargy).

• **Treatment:** Strangulated hernias require emergency surgery to prevent damage to the trapped tissue and restore normal blood flow. This condition can be life-threatening if not treated promptly.

Managing Pediatric Hernias

1. When to Seek Medical Attention

• If you notice a bulge in your child's abdomen or groin, especially if it becomes more pronounced when they cry, strain, or cough, it's important to seek medical advice. While some hernias may resolve on their own (like umbilical hernias in infants), others may require surgery, especially if they cause pain or complications.

2. **Surgical Intervention**

• **Why It's Often Necessary:** While some pediatric hernias, like umbilical hernias, may close on their own, many require surgical repair to prevent complications such as incarceration or strangulation. Inguinal hernias, for example, will not resolve without surgical intervention.

• **What to Expect:** Surgery for pediatric hernias is typically performed under general anesthesia, and recovery times vary depending on the type of hernia and the child's age. In most cases, children recover quickly, although parents should follow post-surgery care instructions to ensure proper healing and avoid complications.

3. **Long-Term Outlook**

• Most children who undergo hernia surgery recover fully and can return to normal activities within a few weeks. With prompt treatment, the risks of recurrence are low. It's important to maintain follow-up appointments with your pediatrician or surgeon to ensure that the hernia does not return and that the child's abdominal wall is healing properly.

Hernias in Athletes

Athletes, particularly those involved in high-intensity sports or activities that require heavy lifting, running, or twisting movements, are at an increased risk for developing certain types of hernias. While physical activity is essential for overall health and fitness, it can also place significant strain on the abdominal muscles and connective tissues, contributing to the formation of hernias. Understanding how hernias develop in athletes, how to prevent them, and how to manage them when they occur is crucial for maintaining both short-term performance and long-term health.

Prevention of Hernias in Athletes

1. **Core Strengthening and Stability**

   • **Why It's Important:** A strong, stable core is essential for every athlete, as it supports almost every movement and helps absorb the impact forces placed on the body during sports. Weak or imbalanced core muscles can leave athletes vulnerable to hernias, particularly in the groin or abdominal areas.

   • **How to Strengthen:** Athletes should incorporate exercises that target both the deep and superficial muscles of the core, including the transverse abdominis, rectus abdominis, and obliques. Effective exercises include planks, leg raises, and stability ball exercises. Pilates and yoga can also help improve core stability while promoting flexibility.

   • **Balanced Routine:** Core exercises should be balanced with exercises targeting the lower back and hips to ensure overall stability. Avoiding an over-reliance on any one muscle group will help maintain the integrity of the abdominal wall and reduce injury risk.

2. **Proper Technique and Form**

• **Why It's Important:** Poor technique during exercises or sports activities increases the risk of injury. When athletes use improper form, they may put unnecessary pressure on the abdominal region, especially during heavy lifting, sprinting, or quick direction changes.

• **Correct Lifting Form:** When lifting weights, athletes should focus on maintaining a neutral spine and engage the core to stabilize the torso. Squats, deadlifts, and other heavy lifting movements should be done with proper alignment and gradual progression in weight.

• **Avoiding Sudden Movements:** Many sports require rapid movements, such as sprinting or pivoting, which can place added pressure on the abdominal area. Athletes should train for quick acceleration and deceleration with proper mechanics to reduce unnecessary strain on the body.

3. **Gradual Training Progression**

• **Why It's Important:** Athletes who jump into intense physical activity without proper conditioning are at risk of overloading their abdominal muscles and connective tissues, which can lead to a hernia. Gradually increasing intensity allows the body to adjust to the demands of the sport.

• **How to Implement:** Start with a solid foundation of fitness, including strength, flexibility, and endurance, before progressing to higher-impact activities. This will help the body adapt and minimize the risk of injury.

• **Rest and Recovery:** Adequate rest is a crucial part of any training program. Overuse or training through pain can lead to muscle imbalances and weaknesses that contribute to hernia formation. Ensure proper rest between workouts and listen to the body to avoid pushing beyond physical limits.

4. **Stretching and Flexibility**

• **Why It's Important:** Tight muscles, particularly in the lower back, hips, and groin, can create imbalances and places of tension in the abdominal wall, increasing the risk of strain and hernia formation. Regular stretching helps maintain muscle length and flexibility, reducing tightness that can lead to injury.

• **How to Stretch:** Incorporate dynamic stretching during warm-ups and static stretching during cool-downs. Focus on the hip flexors, hamstrings, and lower back to promote flexibility. Hip mobility exercises can also be beneficial in preventing groin injuries and reducing stress on the abdominal wall.

5. **Proper Nutrition**

• **Why It's Important:** Nutrition plays a role in muscle function and recovery. Inadequate nutrition or dehydration can lead to muscle weakness or fatigue, which may increase the risk of injury and hernia development.

• **What to Focus On:** Ensure adequate protein intake to support muscle growth and repair, as well as healthy fats and carbohydrates to fuel training. Hydration is essential for muscle function, so be sure to drink plenty of water throughout the day.

• **Supplements:** While a balanced diet is the best source of nutrients, some athletes may benefit from supplements such as vitamin D, magnesium, or omega-3 fatty acids, which support muscle function and recovery. Always consult with a healthcare provider before starting any new supplementation.

Management of Hernias in Athletes

Despite the best efforts at prevention, athletes may still develop hernias due to the physical demands of their sports. Prompt diagnosis and appropriate management are essential to avoid long-term damage and maintain athletic performance.

1. **Recognizing the Symptoms of a Hernia**

   • **Common Symptoms in Athletes:** Inguinal hernias, the most common type for athletes, typically present as a bulge or swelling in the groin area, especially when the athlete strains or engages in physical activity. There may also be discomfort or a dull ache in the affected area.

   • **Red Flags:** Severe pain, nausea, vomiting, or a noticeable bulge that cannot be pushed back into place may indicate a more serious condition, such as an incarcerated or strangulated hernia. These require immediate medical attention.

2. **Non-Surgical Management (For Minor Cases)**

   • **Rest and Activity Modification:** In the early stages of a hernia, rest and modification of activities can sometimes alleviate symptoms. Reducing physical activity that involves heavy lifting, running, or twisting may allow the hernia to be managed without surgery, though this depends on the severity of the condition.

- **Support Garments:** Athletes may use a supportive truss or hernia belt to help alleviate discomfort and support the abdominal wall during light physical activity. However, these devices are not a long-term solution and should not be relied upon for heavy training or competition.

3. **Surgical Intervention**

- **When Surgery is Needed:** Surgery is often the best option for athletes with moderate to severe hernias, especially if the hernia causes significant pain or interferes with athletic performance. The goal of surgery is to repair the tear or weakness in the abdominal wall and prevent the hernia from recurring.

- **Surgical Approaches:** The most common method for repairing hernias is through laparoscopic surgery, which involves small incisions and a quicker recovery time. For some athletes, open surgery may be necessary depending on the type and location of the hernia.

- **Timing the Surgery:** Athletes who require surgery should plan it during the off-season or a time when they can take time off from their sport to recover. Recovery time will vary depending on the severity of the hernia and the surgical approach, but most athletes can return to full activity within 6-12 weeks.

4. **Post-Surgery Rehabilitation**

- **Rehabilitation:** After surgery, athletes will need to follow a structured rehabilitation program to regain strength and flexibility, particularly in the abdominal area. Physical therapy is often recommended to guide the athlete through safe, gradual movements and exercises to rebuild core strength.

- **Gradual Return to Sport:** Athletes should not rush back into intense physical activity after surgery. A gradual return to sport ensures that the abdominal muscles and tissues are fully healed and that the risk of re-injury or recurrence is minimized.

- **Ongoing Strengthening:** Even after surgery, continuing core strengthening exercises and proper movement patterns are essential for long-term health. Athletes should incorporate exercises that focus on both prevention and performance, as a strong core is key for injury-free athleticism.

Hernias in Women

While hernias are often thought of as conditions affecting primarily men, women can also develop hernias, and they may experience unique challenges related to their gender-specific anatomy and life events, such as pregnancy. Understanding the different ways hernias manifest in women, as well as the specific considerations for managing and preventing them, is crucial for providing effective care and treatment.

Pregnancy and Hernias

Pregnancy is a time of significant physical changes, including increased pressure on the abdominal wall. As the baby grows, the body undergoes adaptations that can influence the likelihood of developing a hernia. Women who are pregnant are at increased risk for certain types of hernias due to the mechanical and hormonal changes that occur during this time.

1. **Increased Abdominal Pressure**

    • **How It Happens:** As the pregnancy progresses, the growing uterus puts increasing pressure on the abdominal wall and organs. This constant pressure can weaken the muscles and fascia of the abdomen, making them more susceptible to hernias, especially in the later stages of pregnancy.

    • **Common Hernia Types in Pregnancy:** The most common hernias in pregnant women are **inguinal hernias** (in the groin) and **umbilical hernias** (around the belly button). Umbilical hernias, in particular, are often more pronounced during pregnancy as the increased abdominal pressure exacerbates any existing weakness in the umbilical region.

2. **Inguinal Hernias in Pregnancy**

    • **How They Develop:** Inguinal hernias in women are less common than in men, but pregnancy can increase the risk. As the uterus grows, the pressure in the abdominal cavity can force part of the intestine through the inguinal canal, leading to an inguinal hernia. While this type of hernia is more frequent in men, women can experience it as well, especially during the later stages of pregnancy.

    • **Symptoms and Management:** Pregnant women with inguinal hernias may notice a bulge in the groin, especially when coughing or straining. The hernia may become more noticeable during pregnancy due to the increased abdominal pressure. Most women can manage mild cases with rest, avoiding heavy lifting, and wearing a supportive garment, but surgery is often recommended after pregnancy if the hernia does not resolve.

3. **Umbilical Hernias in Pregnancy**

• **How They Develop:** During pregnancy, the abdominal muscles stretch to accommodate the growing fetus, which can cause weakness in the umbilical region. In some cases, a portion of the intestine or fat may push through the abdominal wall near the belly button, resulting in an umbilical hernia.

• **Symptoms:** Women with umbilical hernias during pregnancy may notice a bulge around the belly button, which may become more pronounced when straining or laughing. Although the bulge may reduce or disappear after childbirth, in some cases, surgery may be needed if the hernia persists.

• **Management:** Many women find that their umbilical hernia becomes less noticeable after childbirth as the abdominal wall regains some of its pre-pregnancy tone. However, if the hernia causes pain or remains visible, surgical repair may be necessary.

4. **Strangulated or Incarcerated Hernias**

• **How They Happen:** Although rare, a hernia can become incarcerated or strangulated, meaning the tissue becomes trapped and the blood supply is cut off. This is a medical emergency, and if a pregnant woman experiences symptoms such as severe pain, vomiting, and a bulging hernia that cannot be pushed back in, immediate medical attention is required.

• **Management:** Strangulated hernias require surgery, and the timing will depend on the stage of pregnancy. In some cases, surgery may be performed during the pregnancy if the hernia poses a risk to the woman's health or the pregnancy itself, though the decision must be made carefully in consultation with the obstetrician and surgeon.

Gender-Specific Considerations for Women and Hernias

While hernias can affect anyone, women may face unique factors that influence the occurrence, management, and treatment of hernias. These factors include differences in anatomy, hormonal fluctuations, and pregnancy-related changes, which can all affect how hernias develop and how they are treated.

1. **Anatomical Differences**

   • **Abdominal Wall and Pelvic Floor:** Women generally have a wider pelvis and different pelvic floor structures compared to men. This anatomical difference affects how the abdominal wall functions and how pressure is distributed throughout the abdomen. Women may be more likely to experience certain types of hernias, such as **incisional hernias** after abdominal surgery, due to these structural differences.

   • **Inguinal Canal:** Although inguinal hernias are more common in men, women can develop them as well. The inguinal canal in women contains the round ligament of the uterus, which is smaller and less prone to injury than the spermatic cord in men. However, this area is still a potential site for hernias, particularly in the context of increased abdominal pressure, such as during pregnancy.

2. **Hormonal Fluctuations**

• **Impact on Connective Tissue:** Hormonal changes, particularly during pregnancy and menopause, can influence the elasticity and strength of connective tissues. The hormone **relaxin**, which is produced during pregnancy to allow the pelvis to widen for childbirth, can also affect the abdominal muscles, making them more prone to strain and hernias.

• **Post-Menopausal Considerations:** After menopause, the decrease in estrogen can lead to a reduction in collagen production, potentially making the abdominal wall less resilient and more susceptible to hernias, particularly in women who are overweight or have a history of abdominal surgeries.

3. **Surgical History**

• **Incisional Hernias:** Women who have had previous abdominal surgeries, such as C-sections or hysterectomies, may be at higher risk for developing **incisional hernias**. These occur when a weakness develops in the abdominal wall at the site of a previous incision, and can be exacerbated by pregnancy or weight gain.

• **Pelvic Surgeries:** Other pelvic surgeries, such as those for endometriosis or fibroids, can also increase the risk of hernias in the pelvic area. Women who have had these surgeries should be mindful of any symptoms that could indicate a hernia, such as pain or swelling near the surgical site.

Management of Hernias in Women

1. **Non-Surgical Management**

• In some cases, women with mild hernias, particularly those that develop during pregnancy, can manage their condition through rest and activity modification. Wearing a supportive garment, such as a hernia belt, may help reduce discomfort, especially if the hernia is in the inguinal or umbilical region.

• **Pain Management:** Over-the-counter pain relief, such as acetaminophen, may be used to manage mild discomfort, though it is important to consult with a healthcare provider before taking any medications, especially during pregnancy.

2. **Surgical Management**

• **Timing of Surgery:** Surgery is often recommended for women with hernias that cause significant pain or those that do not resolve after pregnancy. In cases of more severe hernias or complications such as incarceration or strangulation, surgery may be necessary immediately. The type of surgery—whether open or laparoscopic—depends on the hernia's location, size, and the woman's overall health.

• **Post-Surgical Care:** Women who undergo hernia repair surgery will need time to recover, which may involve avoiding strenuous physical activity, especially activities that could strain the abdominal wall, like heavy lifting. Rehabilitation and physical therapy may be recommended to restore core strength and prevent recurrence.

\

Chapter 8: Emotional and Psychological Impact

Dealing with a hernia, whether it's a new diagnosis or managing an ongoing condition, can have a profound emotional and psychological impact. The physical symptoms of a hernia—pain, discomfort, and limitations on daily activities—are often accompanied by emotional challenges. Understanding the emotional responses that can arise and learning how to manage them is a critical aspect of overall recovery. In this chapter, I will explore how hernias can affect mental health, the coping mechanisms that can help, and the importance of support systems.

Coping with Diagnosis

Receiving a diagnosis of a hernia, particularly if it requires surgery or lifestyle changes, can trigger a range of emotional responses. How a person processes this diagnosis varies depending on their circumstances, personality, and support system. It's essential to acknowledge these emotional reactions as a natural part of the experience.

Emotional Responses to Hernia Diagnosis

1. **Shock and Disbelief**

   - **Initial Reactions:** When first diagnosed with a hernia, especially if symptoms have been mild or unnoticeable for a while, many people experience a sense of disbelief. They may not have expected to be dealing with a health issue, or they may feel shocked by the prospect of surgery or long-term management.

• **Why It Happens:** This emotional response often stems from the unexpected nature of the diagnosis and the sudden realization that they must now prioritize their health in a way that might be inconvenient or uncomfortable.

• **How to Cope:** It can help to take time to absorb the information and process it in stages. Seeking clarification from your healthcare provider about the condition, its progression, and treatment options can provide a sense of control and lessen confusion.

2. **Anxiety and Fear**

• **Fear of Surgery:** For many people, the thought of surgery—whether it's invasive or minimally invasive—can trigger anxiety. Concerns about the risks of anesthesia, complications during surgery, or the fear of not being able to return to normal activities after recovery can feel overwhelming.

• **Fear of Recurrence:** There may also be anxiety about the possibility of the hernia recurring after treatment. Many individuals worry about whether lifestyle changes, physical limitations, or future surgeries will be necessary.

• **How to Cope:** Anxiety can be alleviated by gathering information and having open discussions with healthcare professionals. Knowing the risks, benefits, and expected outcomes of treatment options can help reduce fear. Practicing relaxation techniques, such as deep breathing or meditation, can also be beneficial for calming the mind.

3. **Frustration and Helplessness**

    • **Dealing with Limitations:** As hernias can often limit physical activities, especially those that require heavy lifting, running, or other strenuous movements, individuals may feel frustrated by their inability to participate in daily tasks or hobbies. This can lead to feelings of helplessness, particularly if recovery is slow or if the hernia prevents them from engaging in activities they enjoy.

    • **Social Impact:** Hernias, especially those that involve visible bulges or discomfort in the abdominal area, can also affect self-esteem and body image. This may result in embarrassment or a reluctance to socialize, further intensifying feelings of isolation and frustration.

    • **How to Cope:** Acknowledging the frustration and allowing oneself to feel these emotions is an important step. It's also helpful to work on redefining what physical activity and well-being mean during recovery. Finding alternative exercises or hobbies that don't exacerbate symptoms can help maintain a sense of accomplishment and prevent a total loss of routine. Emotional support from friends, family, or mental health professionals can provide an outlet for these feelings.

4. **Depression and Isolation**

    • **Impact on Mental Health:** Chronic pain, limited mobility, and the fear of ongoing health issues can lead to feelings of sadness, depression, or loneliness. Women and men alike may feel isolated, especially if their social activities are limited by the physical constraints of the hernia.

• **Why It Happens:** The psychological toll of dealing with a medical condition that affects daily life and the possibility of surgery can take a significant emotional toll. Constantly dealing with discomfort or the fear of recurrence can lead to feelings of helplessness or low mood.

• **How to Cope:** If feelings of depression or isolation persist, seeking professional support from a counselor or therapist is essential. Talking to others who have experienced similar conditions, whether through support groups or online communities, can help individuals feel understood and supported.

5. **Acceptance and Adjustment**

• **Adapting to Life with a Hernia:** Over time, many people find that they can come to terms with the limitations a hernia may place on their life, especially with treatment or surgery. Acceptance doesn't mean giving up on recovery or improvement but finding a balanced approach to managing the condition while adjusting expectations.

• **Building Resilience:** As the recovery process progresses, individuals often develop greater resilience, learning how to live with a hernia in a way that minimizes its impact on their lifestyle. This might involve accepting certain physical limitations while still focusing on enjoying life and maintaining overall health.

• **How to Cope:** Acceptance involves acknowledging the reality of the situation and making peace with it. Engaging in mindfulness practices, such as meditation or yoga, can help individuals find balance and reduce the emotional weight of living with a hernia.

Support Systems and Mental Health Strategies

One of the most important factors in coping with the emotional and psychological impact of a hernia diagnosis is a strong support system. Both emotional and practical support from family, friends, and healthcare providers can make a significant difference in how individuals handle their condition.

1. **Family and Friends**

   • **The Role of Loved Ones:** Having a network of supportive family members and friends is invaluable during this time. They can help with day-to-day tasks, provide emotional reassurance, and offer encouragement during recovery. It's also important for loved ones to understand the emotional impact of the condition and be there to listen when needed.

   • **How to Foster Support:** Open communication is key. Expressing needs and feelings clearly can help loved ones understand how best to offer support. It's also helpful to allow others to provide help when needed, as some people feel uncomfortable asking for assistance.

2. **Healthcare Providers**

   • **The Role of Doctors and Therapists:** Physicians, especially those with experience in hernia treatment, can provide not only medical care but also reassurance and clarity regarding the condition. A doctor who takes the time to explain the condition and the treatment options can reduce fear and uncertainty.

• **Mental Health Professionals:** For individuals experiencing significant anxiety, depression, or frustration, seeking the support of a counselor or therapist can be incredibly beneficial. Cognitive-behavioral therapy (CBT) is particularly effective in helping individuals reframe negative thoughts and cope with the emotional challenges of dealing with a health condition.

3. **Support Groups and Online Communities**

• **Connecting with Others:** Many people find comfort in connecting with others who are facing similar challenges. Online support groups or in-person support groups for individuals with hernias can provide a sense of community and understanding. These groups can be a valuable resource for sharing experiences, tips, and coping strategies.

• **Peer Support:** Peer support can alleviate feelings of isolation and encourage individuals to continue their recovery journey. Hearing from others who have overcome the same challenges can inspire hope and help set realistic expectations for what recovery will look like.

4. **Mental Health Strategies**

• **Mindfulness and Meditation:** Techniques such as mindfulness, yoga, and meditation can help individuals manage stress and emotional pain associated with a hernia. These practices promote relaxation, focus, and emotional balance, helping to reduce anxiety and improve overall mental well-being.

• **Journaling:** Writing down thoughts, frustrations, and fears can be an effective way to process emotions and track progress during recovery. Journaling can also help individuals gain perspective on their journey and celebrate small victories along the way.

• **Physical Activity:** Gentle exercises that don't exacerbate hernia symptoms, such as walking or swimming, can improve both physical and mental well-being. Exercise helps release endorphins, the body's natural mood boosters, which can help alleviate feelings of depression and improve overall energy levels.

Living with a Hernia

Living with a hernia presents a unique set of challenges, both physically and emotionally. Whether you're managing a small, asymptomatic hernia or recovering from surgery, it's important to adapt your lifestyle in a way that accommodates the condition while still allowing you to live a full and fulfilling life. In this section, we'll explore the adjustments that many people with hernias make in their daily routines, as well as share inspirational stories from individuals who have successfully managed their hernias and continued to lead active, meaningful lives.

Adjusting to Lifestyle Changes

Living with a hernia often requires modifying certain aspects of your life, but these adjustments can lead to healthier, more balanced habits that benefit both your physical and emotional well-being. While it can feel overwhelming at first, these changes can help prevent worsening symptoms, minimize the risk of complications, and improve your overall quality of life.

1. **Physical Activity Modifications**

    • **Gentle Exercises:** One of the most important lifestyle adjustments involves adapting your exercise routine to protect the hernia and avoid straining the abdominal wall. This may mean switching from high-impact exercises, such as running or heavy lifting, to gentler activities like walking, swimming, or cycling. These low-impact exercises keep you active without exacerbating the hernia.

    • **Strengthening Core Muscles:** While certain exercises may need to be avoided, strengthening the muscles around the hernia, particularly the core, can provide support to the weakened area. This can reduce discomfort and help protect against further damage. A physical therapist can recommend appropriate exercises that target these muscles safely.

    • **Avoiding Strain:** Activities that involve lifting heavy objects or strenuous physical labor should be minimized. Lifting techniques that avoid straining, such as bending at the knees and keeping the back straight, are key to preventing further injury. Many people find that taking frequent breaks or asking for help when moving heavy objects makes a huge difference in their comfort level.

2. **Dietary Adjustments**

    • **Avoiding Constipation:** If you have a hernia, particularly a hiatal or inguinal hernia, constipation can worsen symptoms by putting additional pressure on the abdominal wall. Eating a high-fiber diet and drinking plenty of water can help keep digestion smooth and prevent constipation. Foods rich in fiber, such as fruits, vegetables, and whole grains, can promote regular bowel movements and reduce the risk of straining.

• **Anti-Inflammatory Diet:** An anti-inflammatory diet—rich in fruits, vegetables, lean proteins, and healthy fats—can help reduce any underlying inflammation and support the healing of the abdominal tissues. For those managing hernias, an anti-inflammatory approach can also reduce discomfort associated with the condition.

• **Smaller, More Frequent Meals:** For those with hiatal hernias, particularly those who experience heartburn or acid reflux, eating smaller, more frequent meals throughout the day rather than large meals can reduce pressure on the stomach and ease symptoms.

3. **Mindful Lifestyle Choices**

• **Stress Management:** Chronic stress can contribute to physical tension, which might exacerbate hernia symptoms or delay recovery. Mindfulness techniques such as meditation, deep breathing exercises, and yoga can help reduce stress and improve overall well-being. Incorporating relaxation into daily life is especially important for those managing a chronic condition.

• **Prioritizing Sleep:** Getting adequate rest and sleep is critical for recovery and overall health. For those recovering from hernia surgery, proper sleep helps the body heal and reduces inflammation. Creating a restful sleep environment and developing a bedtime routine can enhance the quality of sleep.

• **Posture and Body Mechanics:** Proper posture is essential when living with a hernia. Slouching or poor posture can place added strain on the abdominal wall. Simple adjustments like sitting upright with support, avoiding excessive bending, and standing tall can reduce the pressure on the hernia and prevent worsening symptoms.

4. **Self-Care and Monitoring**

• **Regular Check-ups:** For those living with a hernia, especially if it's not surgically repaired, it's essential to keep up with regular check-ups to monitor the condition and ensure it isn't worsening. Regular visits to your healthcare provider can help you stay on track with any necessary treatments or lifestyle adjustments.

• **Wearing Support Garments:** Some individuals with hernias find it helpful to wear a supportive garment, such as a hernia belt or truss, to relieve pressure and reduce discomfort. These garments help by holding the hernia in place and supporting the abdominal wall, especially during physical activity.

• **Listening to Your Body:** It's essential to be mindful of any changes in symptoms. If a hernia becomes more painful, enlarges, or causes other complications, it's important to seek medical attention. Being proactive about health and staying attuned to your body's signals can prevent serious complications and improve overall outcomes.

Inspirational Stories from Individuals with Hernias

Living with a hernia doesn't mean you have to sacrifice your goals, dreams, or active lifestyle. Many people with hernias have successfully adapted to their condition and continue to live full, healthy lives. Their stories can serve as a powerful source of inspiration and a reminder that it's possible to thrive, even when faced with challenges.

1. **Sarah's Story: Overcoming the Limitations of an Inguinal Hernia**

    • **Background:** Sarah, a 38-year-old teacher, was diagnosed with an inguinal hernia after noticing a small bulge in her lower abdomen. At first, she was scared and frustrated, thinking it would stop her from being able to exercise and stay active. She was especially worried about the impact it would have on her work life and her ability to care for her young children.

    • **Journey:** After consulting with her doctor, Sarah made the decision to avoid surgery for the time being and focused on modifying her lifestyle. She began incorporating gentle stretching, walking, and core strengthening exercises into her routine. With guidance from a physical therapist, she learned how to strengthen her abdominal muscles safely and reduce the strain on her hernia. Sarah also made dietary changes to prevent constipation and ease her symptoms.

    • **Outcome:** Sarah's hernia symptoms gradually improved as she adapted her lifestyle. Although she still wears a supportive belt during exercise, she is now able to continue running and playing with her kids without significant discomfort. Her story highlights how lifestyle adjustments, exercise modifications, and patience can lead to a successful and fulfilling life despite a hernia diagnosis.

2. **James' Story: Managing a Hiatal Hernia and Finding Peace**

- **Background:** James, a 52-year-old accountant, had been struggling with a hiatal hernia for years, dealing with frequent acid reflux and occasional chest pain. He initially found it difficult to accept the diagnosis and was concerned about the limitations it would place on his work and social life.

- **Journey:** After seeing a specialist, James made significant lifestyle changes, including eating smaller, more frequent meals and cutting out foods that aggravated his symptoms. He also began practicing yoga to improve his posture and reduce stress, which had been contributing to his symptoms. With his doctor's guidance, James learned to listen to his body and avoid triggers that could make his condition worse.

- **Outcome:** Over time, James' symptoms became more manageable, and he found himself less focused on his hernia. He was able to resume his regular activities, including hiking with friends and attending family events without feeling limited. His story is a testament to the power of lifestyle modifications, patience, and emotional resilience in overcoming the challenges of living with a hernia.

3. **Maria's Story: Returning to Active Living After Hernia Surgery**

- **Background:** Maria, a 45-year-old marathon runner, was devastated when she was diagnosed with an inguinal hernia just a few months before a major race she had been training for. The thought of giving up her passion for running and fitness was overwhelming, but she was determined not to let the hernia control her life.

• **Journey:** After consulting with a surgeon, Maria decided to have surgery to repair the hernia. Following the procedure, she focused on a gradual recovery plan, beginning with gentle walks and stretching exercises. She worked closely with a physical therapist to ensure that her abdominal muscles healed correctly and that she wouldn't put undue stress on the area during her recovery.

• **Outcome:** Within a year, Maria was back to running and had even completed the marathon she had been training for before her diagnosis. Her story illustrates that, with the right care and a gradual, thoughtful approach to recovery, it's possible to return to an active lifestyle after surgery and continue pursuing your passions.

Chapter 9: Innovations and Research

In the world of healthcare, innovation is constant. Advances in hernia treatment have improved the lives of millions by making diagnosis faster, treatment more effective, and recovery quicker. As the field of hernia management continues to evolve, cutting-edge technologies, minimally invasive techniques, and new insights from ongoing research are paving the way for improved outcomes. This chapter will explore the latest advancements in hernia treatment, focusing on innovations that are shaping the future of care for individuals with this condition.

Advances in Treatment

In recent years, there have been significant strides in both surgical and non-surgical approaches to hernia treatment. These advancements aim to minimize recovery times, reduce risks of recurrence, and enhance patient comfort. Let's look at some of the most promising innovations and research findings in hernia management.

1. Minimally Invasive Surgery

Minimally invasive surgery, especially laparoscopic and robotic-assisted procedures, has transformed the way hernias are repaired. These techniques allow for smaller incisions, reduced scarring, less post-operative pain, and faster recovery times compared to traditional open surgery.

• **Laparoscopic Hernia Repair:** Laparoscopy involves making a few small incisions and using a camera (laparoscope) to guide the surgeon in repairing the hernia. This approach is increasingly used for various types of hernias, including inguinal, umbilical, and even hiatal hernias. The key benefits include faster recovery, minimal scarring, and a lower risk of infection.

• **Robotic-Assisted Surgery:** A more advanced form of minimally invasive surgery, robotic-assisted hernia repair involves using a robotic system to perform highly precise movements. This approach allows surgeons to work in tight spaces with enhanced control, leading to fewer complications and potentially lower rates of recurrence. While robotic surgery requires specialized equipment and training, its growing availability is a game-changer in hernia treatment.

• **Benefits of Minimally Invasive Approaches:**

• **Reduced Post-Surgery Pain:** Because the incisions are smaller, there's less trauma to the surrounding tissue, which results in less pain after the procedure.

• **Shorter Recovery Time:** Patients who undergo minimally invasive surgery can often return to work and normal activities within a few days to a few weeks, depending on the type of hernia and the specific surgery.

• **Lower Risk of Complications:** Minimally invasive techniques tend to have a lower risk of wound infections, bleeding, and hernia recurrence when compared to traditional methods.

2. Tissue Engineering and Biologic Meshes

Traditional hernia repair involves the use of synthetic mesh to reinforce the abdominal wall and prevent recurrence. However, ongoing research is exploring the use of biologic and tissue-engineered meshes that could offer even better results.

• **Biologic Meshes:** Made from animal tissues (usually pig or cow), biologic meshes are used to repair hernias, especially in cases where traditional synthetic meshes are not recommended due to infection risk or complications. Biologic meshes are designed to be gradually absorbed by the body as natural tissue grows over them, reducing the risk of long-term foreign body reactions.

• **Tissue-Engineered Meshes:** Researchers are also developing tissue-engineered meshes made from human cells that are capable of growing and integrating with the body more seamlessly. These meshes have the potential to provide a more natural repair with fewer complications and a lower recurrence rate. Tissue-engineered meshes are still in the experimental stages but hold great promise for the future of hernia surgery.

• **Improved Healing and Reduced Recurrence:** Biologic and tissue-engineered meshes may promote better integration with the body's own tissues and improve healing, especially in patients with complex hernias or those who are at high risk of complications. These materials are designed to minimize the body's immune response, which may reduce the likelihood of infections and the chance of hernia recurrence.

3. Enhanced Recovery After Surgery (ERAS) Protocols

Enhanced Recovery After Surgery (ERAS) is a multi-disciplinary approach aimed at improving the surgical experience and recovery process for patients. While ERAS protocols have been applied to many types of surgeries, their use in hernia surgery has shown particularly promising results.

- **What ERAS Involves:** ERAS protocols focus on optimizing several aspects of the surgical process, including preoperative nutrition, pain management, and early mobilization after surgery. This holistic approach helps reduce complications, shorten hospital stays, and accelerate recovery.

- **Key Components of ERAS for Hernia Surgery:**

  - **Preoperative Education:** Patients are educated about the surgery and recovery process in advance, reducing anxiety and improving outcomes.

  - **Optimized Pain Management:** Multimodal pain management techniques, which combine various medications and approaches, are used to minimize the use of opioids, reduce pain, and promote quicker recovery.

  - **Early Mobilization:** Encouraging patients to begin walking and performing light activities as soon as possible after surgery reduces the risk of complications like blood clots and helps the body heal faster.

- **Results:** Studies have shown that ERAS protocols for hernia surgery significantly reduce recovery time and improve patient satisfaction. Many patients who follow ERAS guidelines can be discharged within 24 hours of surgery and return to normal activities much sooner than traditional recovery methods allow.

4. Artificial Intelligence and 3D Imaging for Diagnosis and Surgery

Artificial intelligence (AI) and 3D imaging are rapidly transforming the diagnostic and surgical landscape for hernia care. These technologies are helping healthcare providers make more accurate diagnoses, plan surgical procedures more precisely, and enhance the patient experience.

• **AI in Diagnosis:** AI-powered algorithms can analyze imaging results (such as CT scans or MRIs) to identify hernias with a high degree of accuracy. This technology can detect even the smallest hernias that might be missed by the human eye, leading to earlier diagnoses and more targeted treatment plans.

• **3D Imaging for Surgery:** Surgeons are using 3D imaging technologies to better visualize hernias and the surrounding tissues during surgery. With 3D models of a patient's anatomy, surgeons can plan and execute the repair with greater precision. This is especially useful for complex hernias or cases where the hernia is located in difficult-to-reach areas.

• **Benefits of AI and 3D Imaging:**

  • **More Accurate Diagnoses:** AI improves the accuracy of detecting and diagnosing hernias, especially in challenging cases.

  • **Customized Treatment Plans:** With the help of 3D imaging, surgeons can create more personalized treatment plans that take into account the specific anatomical features of the patient.

- **Improved Surgical Outcomes:** The precision afforded by AI and 3D imaging technologies can lead to better surgical outcomes, reduced complications, and faster recovery.

5. Focus on Non-Surgical Alternatives

While surgery remains the primary treatment for most hernias, ongoing research into non-surgical alternatives has led to the development of new methods that may be appropriate for certain patients.

- **Hernia Trusses and Belts:** For individuals who are not candidates for surgery or who prefer to delay surgery, hernia trusses and support belts are being continually improved. These devices are designed to support the hernia and reduce symptoms by holding the protruding tissue in place.

- **Injections and Biologics:** New treatments, such as the injection of biologic substances that promote tissue regeneration or the use of collagen-stimulating injections, are being explored as potential non-surgical options for managing hernias, particularly for those with smaller or less symptomatic hernias.

- **Benefits of Non-Surgical Options:** Non-surgical treatments can be beneficial for individuals who are unable to undergo surgery due to other medical conditions or for those who are seeking to avoid surgery for personal reasons. While not a permanent solution, these treatments can provide relief and help manage the condition in the short term.

Future Directions

The field of hernia treatment is on the cusp of exciting transformations, as emerging technologies and innovative techniques continue to evolve. As medical research progresses, new approaches promise to revolutionize how hernias are diagnosed, treated, and managed. In this section, we will explore the future directions of hernia care, highlighting cutting-edge technologies and research that have the potential to significantly improve patient outcomes in the years to come.

1. Genetic Research and Personalized Medicine

Genetic research is playing an increasingly important role in understanding why some individuals are more prone to developing hernias than others. By identifying genetic predispositions, we could see the development of personalized treatments that cater to an individual's unique genetic makeup, allowing for more targeted and effective interventions.

• **Genetic Testing:** Research is underway to identify specific genes that may increase the risk of developing certain types of hernias. For example, variations in genes related to collagen production and tissue strength might make an individual more susceptible to abdominal or inguinal hernias. Genetic testing could eventually help doctors predict who is at higher risk for hernias and offer preventive measures before a hernia develops.

• **Personalized Treatment Plans:** In the future, treatments for hernias could be customized based on a patient's genetic profile. This could involve selecting the most effective surgical approach, tailoring the use of biologic or synthetic mesh, or even providing personalized rehabilitation protocols to speed recovery and reduce recurrence. Personalized medicine may also improve non-surgical management, offering more precise strategies to manage chronic or asymptomatic hernias.

2. Advancements in Biologic Materials

One of the most exciting areas of hernia treatment is the development of advanced biologic materials, which could offer better outcomes than traditional synthetic meshes. Researchers are focusing on creating biocompatible materials that integrate seamlessly with the body's tissues, reduce the risk of rejection or infection, and enhance the repair process.

- **Self-Healing Meshes:** Future developments in biologic meshes may include self-healing materials, capable of regenerating and repairing themselves over time. These meshes would be made of biodegradable materials that dissolve gradually, allowing the body's own tissues to take over the healing process. This approach could reduce the likelihood of complications and mesh-related issues, such as chronic pain or mesh migration.

- **Tissue Engineering:** Advances in tissue engineering are exploring the creation of entirely new, lab-grown tissues that could be used to repair hernias. For example, researchers are working on growing human tissues in the lab to develop biologic scaffolds that would encourage the body to repair damaged areas naturally. In the future, this could allow for more durable, effective repairs, particularly in patients with complex hernias or those who have had multiple surgeries.

- **Smart Meshes:** "Smart" mesh technology is also on the horizon. These meshes are embedded with sensors that can monitor the healing process in real-time, sending data to a healthcare provider. This could allow doctors to track recovery progress more accurately, detect complications early, and adjust treatment plans as needed.

3. Enhanced Robotic-Assisted Surgery

The use of robotics in surgery has already improved hernia repair outcomes, but as technology continues to advance, we can expect even more refined and precise techniques. Enhanced robotic-assisted surgery promises to make procedures even more efficient, with the potential for faster recovery, less risk of complications, and fewer long-term issues.

•   **Greater Precision and Control:** Future robotic systems will likely offer even greater levels of precision and control, enabling surgeons to repair hernias with fewer incisions and less disruption to surrounding tissues. These systems may be able to perform even more complex hernia repairs that are difficult or impossible with current methods.

•   **AI Integration:** As artificial intelligence (AI) technology continues to develop, it will likely be integrated into robotic surgery systems. AI can assist surgeons in making real-time decisions during surgery, such as adjusting for variations in anatomy or optimizing the placement of mesh. AI-powered systems may also be able to predict surgical outcomes based on patient data, allowing for more personalized care and better results.

•   **Expanded Use of Minimally Invasive Techniques:** Robotic-assisted surgery is expected to become even more widely available for patients with different types of hernias, including complex cases. As these systems become more accessible and cost-effective, more healthcare facilities will adopt them, making high-quality, minimally invasive surgeries available to a broader range of patients.

4. Advances in Imaging and Diagnostic Technologies

Early detection of hernias and precise diagnosis are critical to preventing complications and ensuring the most effective treatment. The future holds exciting prospects for new imaging technologies that will make diagnosing hernias faster, more accurate, and non-invasive.

• **AI-Powered Imaging:** AI is increasingly being used to enhance diagnostic imaging for hernias. Machine learning algorithms can analyze medical images, such as CT scans, MRIs, or ultrasounds, to detect hernias with greater accuracy and speed than traditional methods. AI can identify subtle signs of a hernia or its recurrence, even in difficult-to-see areas, allowing doctors to make more accurate diagnoses and treatment decisions.

• **3D Imaging and Augmented Reality:** 3D imaging is already improving the surgical planning process by providing detailed visualizations of the patient's anatomy. In the future, augmented reality (AR) could allow surgeons to visualize the hernia and surrounding tissues in three dimensions during surgery. By overlaying 3D models of a patient's body, AR could assist in making more informed decisions, improving precision, and reducing errors.

• **Non-Invasive Diagnostic Tools:** Research is underway to develop non-invasive diagnostic tools that can detect hernias without requiring traditional imaging techniques. For example, researchers are exploring the use of wearable sensors and skin patches that can monitor abdominal pressure and detect changes that indicate a hernia is present. These tools could revolutionize hernia diagnosis, making it more accessible and less burdensome for patients.

5. Regenerative Medicine and Stem Cell Therapy

The field of regenerative medicine, particularly stem cell therapy, holds immense potential for improving hernia treatment and recovery. Stem cells have the ability to regenerate and repair damaged tissues, making them an exciting prospect for treating hernias, especially those that are difficult to repair or have recurred after surgery.

• **Stem Cell Therapy for Tissue Regeneration:** Researchers are exploring the use of stem cells to promote tissue regeneration at the site of a hernia. Stem cells could help repair weakened abdominal walls or damaged connective tissues, leading to stronger, more durable repairs. This treatment could significantly reduce the risk of recurrence, especially in patients with more complex or recurring hernias.

• **Growth Factors and Biologics:** Alongside stem cells, growth factors and biologic agents are being studied for their ability to stimulate tissue healing and regeneration. By encouraging the body's natural healing processes, these treatments may help speed recovery and improve the long-term strength of the repaired tissues.

• **Personalized Regenerative Approaches:** Combining stem cell therapy with personalized medicine may offer even more tailored treatments. Doctors could use a patient's own stem cells to repair their hernia, reducing the risk of rejection or complications. Personalized regenerative treatments may become a key strategy in treating more challenging or chronic hernias.

6. Artificial Intelligence and Predictive Analytics

AI is also poised to transform how we predict and manage hernia recurrence. By analyzing vast amounts of data, AI can help doctors predict which patients are at the highest risk for hernia recurrence or complications after surgery, enabling more proactive treatment and personalized care plans.

•   **Predictive Analytics:** AI-driven predictive models are being developed to assess a patient's risk of recurrence based on factors such as surgical approach, the type of hernia, and post-surgery behaviors. By using these models, healthcare providers can identify high-risk patients and implement preventative measures before complications arise.

•   **Data-Driven Decisions:** With advancements in big data, healthcare providers will be able to make more informed decisions about hernia management. Machine learning algorithms can analyze large datasets from patient histories, surgeries, and outcomes to optimize treatment protocols, reduce recurrence rates, and improve patient satisfaction.

Chapter 10: Personal Stories and Case Studies

One of the most powerful ways to understand the impact of hernias on people's lives is through the personal stories of those who have faced the condition. In this chapter, we will hear firsthand accounts from individuals who have navigated the challenges of living with, treating, and recovering from hernias. We will also explore case studies that shed light on the different types of hernias, treatment options, and outcomes. Additionally, insights from healthcare professionals will help contextualize these personal experiences, offering a deeper understanding of the medical and emotional journey involved in hernia care.

1. Real-Life Accounts of Individuals Dealing with Hernias

Each person's journey with a hernia is unique, shaped by their individual health circumstances, lifestyle, and approach to treatment. In this section, we will share the stories of several individuals who have faced hernias and how they managed their diagnosis, treatment, and recovery.

Case 1: Mark's Struggle with an Inguinal Hernia

Mark, a 42-year-old construction worker, began to notice a bulge in his lower abdomen after years of heavy lifting at work. Initially, he dismissed it as a minor issue, but the discomfort grew over time. After seeking medical advice, he was diagnosed with an inguinal hernia. Mark's experience highlights how an active, physically demanding job can contribute to the development of hernias.

- **Diagnosis:** Mark initially felt embarrassed and reluctant to seek help, fearing it would prevent him from working. However, as the pain increased, he visited his doctor, who performed a physical exam and confirmed the hernia through an ultrasound.

- **Treatment:** Mark was advised to undergo surgery, and he chose a laparoscopic hernia repair, which allowed him to return to work faster. While the surgery was minimally invasive, the recovery was still challenging. He had to refrain from lifting for several weeks, which caused some anxiety about his ability to return to his job.

- **Post-Surgery:** Mark shared that his biggest challenge was adjusting to a new routine during recovery. However, with the support of his family and a positive mindset, he was able to focus on exercises to strengthen his core muscles and prevent recurrence. He is now back at work and has taken measures to lift safely to reduce the risk of another hernia.

Mark's story demonstrates the importance of early diagnosis and treatment. He emphasized how seeking medical help early could prevent the condition from worsening and ensure a smoother recovery process.

Case 2: Susan's Experience with a Hiatal Hernia

Susan, a 55-year-old woman, began experiencing frequent acid reflux and discomfort in her chest. Initially, she thought it was simply indigestion, but when the symptoms persisted, she visited her doctor. An endoscopy revealed that she had a hiatal hernia, a condition where part of her stomach had moved into her chest cavity.

• **Diagnosis:** Susan's diagnosis was unexpected and troubling. She had never considered a hernia to be the cause of her symptoms. After discussing treatment options with her doctor, she was informed that her hiatal hernia could be managed with medication, lifestyle changes, and in some cases, surgery.

• **Treatment:** Susan chose a conservative approach initially, making dietary adjustments and taking medications to control her acid reflux. She learned to eat smaller meals, avoid trigger foods, and elevate the head of her bed to reduce nighttime symptoms. However, when the reflux worsened, her doctor recommended surgery.

• **Surgical Solution:** Susan eventually opted for a laparoscopic Nissen fundoplication, a procedure that repairs the hiatal hernia and prevents reflux. She found the surgery to be highly effective, but the recovery required her to make significant changes to her eating habits and lifestyle. It was a challenging transition, but she now enjoys a much better quality of life.

Susan's journey underscores the complexity of hiatal hernias, especially for those who experience chronic symptoms like acid reflux. Her story shows that while surgery may be necessary for some individuals, lifestyle changes play a crucial role in managing symptoms and promoting long-term health.

Case 3: Daniel's Battle with an Umbilical Hernia

Daniel, a 28-year-old father of two, noticed a small bulge near his belly button after the birth of his second child.

Initially, he thought it was a simple sign of his body adjusting after childbirth, but the bulge didn't go away. After a few months of discomfort, he visited his doctor and was diagnosed with an umbilical hernia.

- **Diagnosis:** Daniel's hernia was discovered through a physical exam. He was surprised to learn that many people have umbilical hernias without experiencing significant symptoms. His hernia wasn't causing pain but was becoming progressively more noticeable. His doctor explained that many people with umbilical hernias live with them without needing surgery, but Daniel opted to explore treatment options.

- **Treatment:** Given that the hernia was not causing severe discomfort, Daniel chose to manage it non-surgically at first. He used a hernia belt for support during physical activities and adjusted his exercise routine to avoid movements that could put pressure on the hernia.

- **Surgery:** Eventually, Daniel's hernia began to affect his daily activities, and he decided to undergo surgery. He opted for laparoscopic repair, which allowed for a quick recovery and minimal scarring. Post-surgery, he was able to resume normal activities within a few weeks.

Daniel's experience highlights the importance of self-care and making informed decisions when it comes to managing less symptomatic hernias. His case demonstrates that even smaller hernias can sometimes lead to challenges, but the right treatment can significantly improve quality of life.

2. Insights from Healthcare Professionals

Hernias may be common, but every case is unique. Healthcare professionals, from surgeons to physical therapists, offer invaluable perspectives on the medical management of hernias. Here, we'll explore the insights of Dr. Emily Turner, a general surgeon specializing in hernia repair, and Sarah Lawson, a physical therapist who helps patients recover from hernia surgery.

Dr. Emily Turner, General Surgeon:

"As a surgeon, I encounter patients with a variety of hernias, and one of the most important things I emphasize is that not all hernias require immediate surgery. In some cases, patients with small, asymptomatic hernias can lead full, healthy lives without surgical intervention. However, it's crucial to monitor the hernia to ensure it doesn't worsen over time."

Dr. Turner shared that early diagnosis is key. "Patients often wait too long to seek help because they don't realize how much a hernia can impact their lives. A proactive approach to treatment, whether it's surgical or conservative, can make all the difference in the long run."

Sarah Lawson, Physical Therapist:

"Post-surgery rehabilitation plays a critical role in a patient's recovery. After hernia repair, patients must focus on strengthening their core muscles to reduce the risk of recurrence. I work with patients to develop customized exercise plans that promote healing, improve flexibility, and enhance overall strength."

Sarah emphasized that many patients underestimate the importance of recovery exercises. "Even after surgery, it's vital to stay active in ways that don't strain the body. Gentle stretching, low-impact cardio, and strength training tailored to the patient's condition can support long-term recovery and prevent future issues."

3. Conclusion

The personal stories and insights shared in this chapter reflect the diverse experiences of individuals living with hernias. From the physical challenges to the emotional journey, each person's experience is different. By sharing these stories, we gain a deeper understanding of how hernias can affect daily life and the many ways people cope with this condition. With the guidance of healthcare professionals and ongoing advancements in hernia treatment, individuals can make informed decisions about their care and find strategies for managing their condition effectively. Through these narratives, we also see the importance of a holistic approach—combining medical intervention, lifestyle adjustments, and emotional support to ensure the best possible outcomes.

Conclusion

In this guide, we have explored the many facets of hernias—what they are, how they develop, and the various ways they can be managed and treated. We've examined the causes, risk factors, and symptoms associated with different types of hernias, as well as the diagnostic tools available to help identify and understand the condition. We've also delved into prevention strategies, treatment options, post-treatment recovery, and the emotional impact of living with a hernia. Through real-life stories and insights from healthcare professionals, we've gained a comprehensive understanding of hernias from both a medical and personal perspective.

Recap of Key Points

• **Understanding Hernias:** A hernia occurs when an organ or tissue pushes through a weak spot in the surrounding muscle or connective tissue. Hernias can develop in various parts of the body, including the abdomen, groin, and diaphragm, and their symptoms can range from mild discomfort to more severe pain.

• **Causes and Risk Factors:** Genetics, lifestyle choices, occupational hazards, and certain medical conditions all play a role in the development of hernias. Recognizing these risk factors can help individuals take proactive steps to reduce their chances of developing one.

• **Symptoms and Diagnosis:** Hernias may present with visible bulges, pain, or discomfort, particularly during physical activity. Early diagnosis is critical, and healthcare professionals use imaging and clinical examinations to identify the presence of a hernia.

• **Prevention and Treatment:** Strengthening core muscles, using proper lifting techniques, and managing chronic conditions are all essential components of prevention. When surgery is necessary, advancements in minimally invasive techniques have made treatment more effective with quicker recovery times.

• **Post-Treatment and Long-Term Management:** Post-surgery care and lifestyle modifications are crucial for ensuring a smooth recovery and reducing the likelihood of recurrence. Regular follow-ups with healthcare providers help track progress and make adjustments to recovery plans as needed.

• **The Emotional and Psychological Impact:** Coping with a hernia, particularly one that requires surgery, can be emotionally challenging. Having a solid support system and seeking professional guidance can make a significant difference in the healing process.

• **Innovations and Future Directions:** The future of hernia treatment is promising, with advancements in genetic research, biologic materials, robotic-assisted surgery, and regenerative medicine offering new, more personalized approaches to care.

Encouragement for Readers to Take Proactive Steps for Their Health

Taking charge of your health is the first step toward preventing and managing hernias. Whether you're currently living with a hernia or want to reduce your risk, the strategies outlined in this guide can help you make informed decisions about your care. Remember, small lifestyle changes—like maintaining a healthy weight, engaging in regular exercise, and practicing proper lifting techniques—can go a long way in supporting your overall health and preventing hernias. If you have any concerns, don't hesitate to consult a healthcare provider for guidance on how to best care for your body and reduce your risk.

By being proactive and informed, you can take control of your health and feel confident in your ability to manage or prevent hernias, allowing you to live a fulfilling and active life.

Resources for Further Information

While this guide provides a wealth of information, there are additional resources available for those who want to learn more about hernias and related health topics. Below are some valuable sources for further reading and support:

1. **American Hernia Society:** www.americanherniasociety.org
A leading organization for hernia research, treatment, and education. It provides valuable resources for both patients and healthcare providers.

2. **National Institute of Diabetes and Digestive and Kidney Diseases (NIDDK):** www.niddk.nih.gov
Offers comprehensive information on various types of hernias, including treatment options and preventive measures.

3. **Mayo Clinic:** www.mayoclinic.org
A trusted resource for health information, including detailed explanations of hernia symptoms, causes, diagnosis, and treatment options.

4. **Hernia Support Groups:**
Connecting with others who have experienced or are currently dealing with hernias can provide emotional support and practical advice. Look for local or online

support groups dedicated to hernia recovery and management.

5. **Your Healthcare Provider:**

For personalized advice and treatment plans, always consult with your healthcare provider. They can offer the best recommendations based on your unique situation.

By utilizing these resources and staying informed, you are taking a critical step in ensuring your health and well-being, both in the short term and for years to come. Keep learning, stay proactive, and take control of your health journey.

Appendices

This section provides additional resources to further support your understanding of hernias and to help guide you on your journey toward health and recovery. Whether you are seeking clarity on medical terms, looking for support networks, or interested in deepening your knowledge through further reading, these appendices offer valuable tools to assist you.

1. Glossary of Medical Terms

Understanding the medical terminology related to hernias can be helpful in navigating your diagnosis and treatment. Here's a list of key terms used in this guide:

- **Abdomen:** The area of the body between the chest and pelvis, containing vital organs such as the stomach, intestines, and liver.

- **Inguinal Hernia:** A hernia that occurs in the inguinal canal in the lower abdomen, often causing a bulge in the groin area.

- **Femoral Hernia:** A hernia that develops in the upper thigh near the groin, more common in women.

- **Umbilical Hernia:** A hernia that occurs at the belly button (umbilicus), often seen in infants or pregnant women.

- **Hiatal Hernia:** A condition where part of the stomach pushes through the diaphragm into the chest cavity, often causing acid reflux or heartburn.

•   **Incisional Hernia:** A hernia that forms at the site of a previous surgical incision or scar.

•   **Laparoscopic Surgery:** A minimally invasive surgical technique that uses small incisions and a camera to perform the operation.

•   **Core Muscles:** The muscles in the abdomen, back, and pelvis that are responsible for stabilizing the body and aiding in movement.

•   **Strangulation:** A complication of hernias where blood flow to the herniated tissue is cut off, leading to tissue death, often requiring emergency surgery.

•   **Protrusion:** The process of an organ or tissue pushing through a weakened area of muscle or connective tissue.

•   **Hernia Belt:** A support garment worn to help manage a hernia, providing additional pressure to prevent further protrusion or discomfort.

2. List of Helpful Resources and Support Groups

Whether you are dealing with a hernia personally or seeking support for a loved one, connecting with others who understand your experience can be invaluable. Below are some helpful resources and support groups dedicated to hernia awareness and recovery:

•   **American Hernia Society:**
Website: www.americanherniasociety.org
This organization offers educational resources, treatment options, and a network for healthcare providers and patients.

•   **HerniaHelp:**
Website: www.herniahelp.org

A nonprofit that provides information on hernia prevention, treatment, and a database of support groups.

- **Hernia Network:**
Website: www.hernianetwork.org
An online community offering support, advice, and resources for people living with hernias, as well as information on surgery and recovery.

- **National Institute of Diabetes and Digestive and Kidney Diseases (NIDDK):**
Website: www.niddk.nih.gov
Provides authoritative information on hernias, their treatment, and prevention strategies.

- **Hernia Support Groups (Online Forums):**
Many online forums, such as those on Reddit and HealthUnlocked, feature communities where individuals share their experiences with hernia surgery and recovery. Search for "hernia support groups" to find a community near you.

- **Local Hospitals and Clinics:**
Many hospitals and medical centers offer support groups or counseling for individuals undergoing hernia treatment or recovery. Check with your healthcare provider for local recommendations.

3. Suggested Reading and References

If you wish to dive deeper into hernia-related topics, the following books, articles, and research papers provide comprehensive and up-to-date information:

- **Books:**

  - **"Hernia: A Comprehensive Guide"** by Dr. Richard F. Smith

A thorough guide to understanding hernias, their causes, symptoms, and treatment options.

- **"The Hernia Handbook"** by Dr. Peter H. B. McKenna

This book provides practical advice for both patients and healthcare providers on managing hernias.

- **"Surgical Techniques in Hernia Repair"** by Dr. Thomas S. D. Wolff

A detailed textbook focused on the latest techniques and innovations in hernia surgery.

- **Articles:**

- **"The Role of Laparoscopic Surgery in Hernia Repair"** published in *The Journal of Minimally Invasive Surgery*

Discusses the benefits and advancements of minimally invasive procedures for hernia treatment.

- **"The Psychological Impact of Hernias and Surgery"** published in *Journal of Patient Care*

An article that explores the emotional and psychological aspects of living with and recovering from hernias.

- **Research Papers:**

- **"Comparative Effectiveness of Mesh vs Non-Mesh Hernia Repair"** in *The Lancet*

An analysis of the outcomes of mesh versus non-mesh surgical repair for various types of hernias.

- **"Genetic Risk Factors for Hernia Development"** in *Nature Reviews Genetics*

An exploration of genetic factors contributing to hernia formation, highlighting the role of inherited traits in predisposition.

- **Websites for Further Information:**

  - **Mayo Clinic - Hernias Overview:**
  www.mayoclinic.org

  - **Healthline - Hernia Resources:**
  www.healthline.com

  - **WebMD - Understanding Hernias:**
  www.webmd.com

These resources, combined with the knowledge you've gained from this guide, should empower you to make informed decisions about hernia prevention, treatment, and recovery. Whether you're seeking medical advice, practical support, or further education, these tools will help you along your journey to better health.

Made in United States
North Haven, CT
16 May 2025

68941375R00075